DISCARD

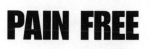

PAIN FREE

BANTAM BOOKS
New York   Toronto   London
Sydney   Auckland

PAIN FREE

A
REVOLUTIONARY METHOD
FOR
STOPPING CHRONIC PAIN

Pete Egoscue DISCARD

with
Roger Gittines

Pacific Grove Public Library

616.0472
EGO

PAIN FREE

A Bantam Book / March 1998

All rights reserved.
Copyright © 1998 by Pete Egoscue.
Photos copyright © The Egoscue Method
Line drawings by Wendy Wray.

No part of this book may be reproduced or transmitted in any form or by any means, electronic
or mechanical, including photocopying, recording, or by any information storage and retrieval
system, without permission in writing from the publisher.
For information address: Bantam Books.

Library of Congress Cataloging-in-Publication Data
Egoscue, Pete, 1945–
Pain free : a revolutionary method for stopping chronic pain / by Peter Egoscue,
with Roger Gittines.
p.   cm.
ISBN 0-553-10630-9
1. Chronic pain—Exercise therapy.   I. Gittines, Roger.   II. Title.
RB127.E35   1998
616′.0472—dc21   97-31745
                                                                          CIP

Published simultaneously in the United States and Canada

Bantam Books are published by Bantam Books, a division of Bantam Doubleday Dell Publishing
Group, Inc. Its trademark, consisting of the words "Bantam Books" and the portrayal of a
rooster, is Registered in U.S. Patent and Trademark Office and in other countries. Marca
Registrada. Bantam Books, 1540 Broadway, New York, New York 10036.

PRINTED IN THE UNITED STATES OF AMERICA
BVG 10 9 8 7 6 5 4 3 2 1

This book is dedicated to my father, Harold Joseph Egoscue, who has lived his life with integrity, purpose, and achievement.

CONTENTS

It has become obligatory for health books to carry a legal disclaimer. You've read them: "The following material is not intended as a substitute for the advice of a physician. . . ." And they go on to recommend that you consult a doctor before embarking on whatever program is being offered. They conclude with the author and publisher disclaiming any legal responsibility for adverse consequences. As I did in my first book, I will again urge readers who feel they need the disclaimer's protection and counsel to close these covers and leave the pages unread. My working principle as an author and exercise therapist is that the most important consultation is the one a person has with him- or herself. Health care starts with personal responsibility. Any disclaimer that suggests otherwise does a great disservice.

LIST OF ILLUSTRATIONS

Chapter 1

Chapter 3

Chapter 4

Chapter 5

Chapter 6

Chapter 7

Chapter 8

Chapter 9

Chapter 10

Chapter 11

Chapter 12

ACKNOWLEDGMENTS

Providing effective therapy to treat chronic musculoskeletal pain and writing a book about it are similar in at least one significant way—they both take teamwork. I will briefly single out a few individuals for special thanks, but it would take pages to express my gratitude adequately. Roger Gittines, whose name is on the cover as my coauthor, also needs to be recognized as a good friend. He worked hard and well to make sure we ended up saying what I meant. Our editor at Bantam Books, Brian Tart, skillfully kept us on track. Brian Bradley, The Egoscue Method Clinic Director, and Erica Lusk, Director of Video Therapy, went above and beyond the call of duty by doing most of the modeling work. The rest of the clinic staff provided great support. Linda and John Lynch, Nevins McBride, Charlie and Vera Richardson, and Alex Quintero made important contributions. Illustrator Wendy Wray proved that while some drawings are worth a thousand words, hers are of a much higher value. Margret McBride, my friend and literary agent, believed in the book and the Method, and never ran out of patience. Finally— saving the most important for last—I'm grateful for all those men and women, girls and boys, who have had the courage to trust their own instincts and their own bodies. They are the real starting lineup for the team that made this book and the Egoscue Method possible.

INTRODUCTION

This is a book about our bodies—yours and mine. We are different in height, weight, and possibly gender. But our common possession is the body's inner power to heal itself and to be pain free. By choosing those two words as my title, I am celebrating our mutual good fortune. I am also making a promise that I know *you* can keep.

Being pain free takes personal effort and commitment. It doesn't come from a pill bottle, a surgeon's knife, a brace, or in specially designed mattresses, chairs, and tools. The thousands of men and women who in the course of a typical year visit my Egoscue Method Clinic in San Diego, California, know it, or they soon find out, and I watch them transform their lives as they rediscover the joy and health that had seemed lost forever. While each client is dedicated to stopping chronic pain in one form or another, they are all taking the easy way out. The easiest, really.

The following pages show you the way. It does not involve high-tech medicine or elaborate physical therapy routines. You won't need to buy special equipment or consult cadres of experts. In the first three chapters, I review how the human body is designed to maintain its own health throughout a *long* lifetime. Episodes of pain are aberrations that can be easily treated if the body is permitted to do its work. Unfortunately, many of us don't understand even the most basic features of this magnificent "machine."

Following this overview are eight chapters, each dealing with a specific chronic pain condition. You have probably already looked at the table of contents. I reverse the usual order and go from foot to head: sore feet, ankles, knees, hips, back, shoulders, elbows, wrists, hands, neck, and head. The chronic pain chapters are set up to give you a quick and thorough briefing on what's happening in that part of the body when it hurts. After each briefing, I offer a series of exercises designed to alleviate the causes of pain in that body part. My friends at the clinic have nicknamed them E-cises, for "Egoscuecises," to tease me for my near obsession with fine-tuning them as therapeutic tools. What started as an inside joke has taken root, and that's what I call them in this book. The E-cises are arranged in menus, and are easy to do and extremely effective. To guide you along, I provide detailed instructions and many photos.

Next comes a chapter on common chronic pain problems relating to popular sports and recreational activities, and finally a concluding chapter that, among other things, offers an overall conditioning menu of E-cises for your use once your chronic pain symptoms abate.

A Quick Guide to Using Pain Free

An author probably should not presume to tell a reader how to read a book, but I will risk it anyway in the interest of making this information as accessible as possible. My guess is that you are in pain or have been in pain recently. Take the time to read the first three chapters, which give you valuable background knowledge. I'll explain how a serious deficiency of "design motion" is causing your chronic pain symptoms and how easy it is for you to remedy the situation. Then quickly flip through the rest of the chapters to get a look at the boxes and breakouts that present key concepts in capsule form. Finally, turn to the chapter that focuses on your specific condition. My hope is that you'll eventually read the book straight through, but I realize that stopping the pain may be paramount in your mind. If I had to choose one additional must-read chapter, it would be chapter 7, which deals with hips. The condition of our hips plays a central role in combating chronic pain throughout the body.

I'll take one more unusual liberty as an author by making this statement: *Pain Free* won't do you much good if you just read it. Information is fine, but action is far better. When practiced both in the clinic and at home, the E-cises in this book yield a ninety-five percent success rate. Yet the Egoscue Method conquers chronic pain only because those who are suffering are empowered with the means to heal themselves—and they use that power. Those among the five percent who are unable to find relief using the Method often do not have the time or the inclination to take action; they do the E-cises sporadically or not at all.

I urge you to use the E-cises. They look simple, but they are calibrated to pinpoint specific musculoskeletal functions that have been compromised by a variety of factors. The E-cise menus are arranged sequentially to address each component of a particular chronic pain symptom. Therefore, you should do the menu in the order it is presented; by picking and choosing E-cises at random, you risk interrupting the sequence. Likewise, if you have active pain, do not shop around in this book for something you think might work. Stick with the menu for the body part where the chronic pain is occurring. If an E-cise is specified for one side of the body, always repeat it on the other side, even though it may be harder or—as is the case many times—it doesn't seem relevant to the pain symptom.

I believe in goal setting and planning. When it comes to managing one's health, the old maxim "Those who do not plan, plan to fail" is particularly true. Even so, people who wouldn't dream of doing business or providing for their families until they had a clear set of objectives and a strategy for achieving them, make major health decisions without knowing what they want, how to realize it, and what the *real* costs will be.

With the Egoscue Method, I ask new clients what they expect to get for their money. Is it pain relief, enhanced athletic performance, or a good night's sleep? There are many legitimate answers. In turn, I tell them what we can do, how much it will cost, how long it will take, and what they will be expected to do. If I don't keep my end of the bargain, the client gets his or her money back. The guarantee is in play from the very first visit. If the client is hurting and doesn't feel better on leaving, the visit is free.

Does this sound like buying an appliance from a reputable dealer, or laying out the terms of an important business deal? Comparisons like that couldn't please me more. Any vendor of health care, mainstream or alternative, who isn't willing to stand by the product must be treated with the utmost caution. They shouldn't hide behind science, expertise, or complexity. If the tough questions aren't asked, shame on you, the consumer; if they're not answered, shame on us, the supplier. Ducking and dodging have the same universal meaning, whether the product comes with four worn tires and suspiciously low mileage or is bristling with terminology that no layperson can understand. As a consumer, the less you know, the more you should worry that the product may not work as advertised. Many common musculoskeletal treatments don't work as advertised; that's why patients find it so difficult to get straight answers to their questions, starting with "Why does it hurt?" They often get *probablies, maybes,* and *chances ares.* Even a direct answer to a question about the cause of joint pain—*cartilage loss*—smothers in a blanket of vagueness when patients ask a follow-up question: "Why is there cartilage loss on the right side and not the left?" When it comes to health care, it is imperative to ask and keep asking the same nuts-and-bolts questions that you would ask in any straightforward consumer transaction.

In addition to being grounded solidly in this consumer-knows-best philosophy, the Egoscue Method's E-cises, by suppressing pain symptoms, eliminate impulses to buy products for which patients probably have no need in the first place. If a surgical procedure or drug regimen is designed to eliminate pain, but exercise therapy has already eliminated it, why bother with the surgery or drugs? "Because," you're likely to be told, "the pain will return." That's correct, it will return. But the most basic question of all is, Why should it return? The answer lies at the heart of the entire Egoscue Method. Unless treatment addresses underlying musculoskeletal dysfunctions, pain relief can be only temporary. Nobody wants to hurt, and nobody should have to. But eliminating the pain symptom is only the first step. Without going to the next one, the muscles will continue to tell the bones to move in ways that violate the body's design. That's why the chronic pain will return.

The only product that's worth investing in is a fully functional musculoskeletal system. It's no luxury but rather a basic necessity that's within everyone's reach.

Pain Free—His Way

Several years ago, I had an appointment to see a prospective new client at a condominium he was using in one of those luxury complexes that have become a standard part of new golf course developments. A tournament was scheduled there, and he was one of the players. When I arrived, the man was coming out his front door at the top of a flight of stairs. He was leaning on the arm of a young man, his oldest son, and was obviously in extreme pain. As I started up the stairs, he noticed me and said, "Sorry to have you come all this distance, Mr. Egoscue. But I'm on my way to withdraw from the tournament. My back is killing me." I said I didn't think it would be necessary and convinced him to wait until after he tried the Method. He was skeptical, but despite the pain, he was a model of patience and courtesy. He turned back to his apartment, helped by his son.

Today, the very weekend that these words are being written, the man, my friend Jack Nicklaus, is playing in his forty-second U.S. Open. He is the oldest player to ever qualify. Jack took action, and he continues to take it every day—as I hope you will.

Not long after our first meeting, Jack Nicklaus noticed a fan following him along as he played in various major tournaments. The fan was very recognizable because of a severe limp; he almost dragged his legs from hole to hole to watch the play. Jack went over to him and gave him my phone number. The fan, Gary, had had a stroke three years before. He came to my clinic after undergoing the standard physical therapy protocol for stroke victims. That protocol usually offers a set number of sessions—often it's six weeks—after which the physical therapist evaluates the patient's physical and mental faculties to determine the extent of permanent damage. At that point, the assumption is that the patient has made all the progress he or she is likely to make. In making this assumption, however, the therapists aren't cruel; they encourage the person to work on their own, but they are eventually discharged and the treatment ends.

This had been Gary's experience. But his walking and balance were still extremely poor, and he still had trouble moving his upper limbs. After three years, even these functions were beginning to deteriorate. He was dying a slow death. When I first met Gary, I asked him if he thought the stroke had caused brain damage. He hesitated, knowing that that is the common diagnosis for a person in his condition. But I encouraged him to answer, and he said emphatically that there had not been brain damage.

"Why can't you move, then?" I asked. All he could do was shrug. I told him to forget the stroke and concentrate on doing the job at hand—restoring musculoskeletal functions that, for whatever reason, had been lost. At the clinic we had him do a set of E-cises: static back presses, knee pillow squeezes, isolated hip flexor lifts (all of them included in this book). His walking quickly improved. The next day, as we talked, I noticed that his hand was clenched in the classic clawlike manner of a stroke victim.

"Open your hand," I said.

"I can't. Haven't for three years."

I gently took him by the arm and raised it over his head. "Now open your hand." And he did.

Gary had more work to do, but he did it and reversed the "permanent" stroke damage.

The point of this story—and of this book—is that we can solve many of these "permanent" problems by refusing to accept the view that age, accidents, or disease routinely triumph over the human body's natural legacy to be pain free.

CHRONIC PAIN: THE MODERN DANGER OF IGNORING AN ANCIENT MESSAGE

The doctors thought I was unconscious—a reasonable assumption in an intensive care ward of a U.S. hospital ship filled with newly arrived Vietnam combat casualties. They stopped at the cot next to mine, where an army captain moaned in agony. He had been shot in the stomach several days before. The soldier was so badly hurt, he never slept, never talked to anyone, never fell into the arms of a merciful silence. There was only the stark, unremitting sound of a human being in pain, punctuated by the beeping of heart monitors.

The doctors looked at his chart and made a brief examination of the massive wound. One of them asked, "Think he'll make it?" I heard the clipboard that held the man's medical record drop back into its holder. I wanted to turn my head to see if they were talking about me, but couldn't manage it. Too many tubes and too much pain of my own.

The other doctor answered with such a matter-of-fact tone that today I imagine him shrugging as he said, "You either get well or you die."

The young captain died a couple of days later. I've been thinking about him and what the doctor said for nearly thirty years. The comment struck me then, as it does now, with the force of a profound truth. The doctor, whether he was aware of it or not, was recognizing that there comes a point when modern medical techniques must give way to the body's own inner logic, mechanisms, and intentions. Despite all the hardware, surgical talent, antibiotics, and pain-killers, you either get well or you die.

This is not fatalism, blind faith, or passivity. It is a confirmation and celebration of the body's capacity to maintain health and life independent of outside intervention that would substitute technology and technical know-how for this ineffable power. Faced with the soldier's agony, the doctor confronted his own limitations. Inadvertently, he allowed me to see that if I was to survive and fully recover from my own wounds, I would have to come to an understanding of why we either get well or do not. As an exercise therapist, a profession I chose as a direct result of the long rehabilitation program that I underwent to return to active duty as a Marine officer, my experience has taught me that the human body not only controls the ultimate transition from life to death but, in the meantime, manages the process that we call health and healing.

Much of what is regarded today as state-of-the-art chronic pain treatment ignores this lesson. An entire industry has developed that replaces hips and knees, that fuses backs and prescribes braces, and that tells patients to take pills and take it easy. The young doctor's comment has been transformed into "Either we make you well or you die." Technology and techniques have become so intrusive that they are usurping the body's own role in health and healing. And that's a tragedy. Ultimately, there can be neither health nor healing if the body is denied its commanding role in making us well.

A Process of Rediscovery

This commanding role starts with the utmost simplicity and strength of the body's design. Its foundation and framework is the musculoskeletal system: muscles, joints, bones, and nerves. I include nerves because the nervous system overlaps and merges functionally with the musculoskeletal system. The interaction of all these components is at once so ingenious, so infinitely complex, and so perfectly suited to the purpose and the material, that any thought of imposing another configuration—no matter how well-intended—should be met with the deepest skepticism. Yet many drastic, highly invasive treatments for chronic pain conditions have become commonplace. These treatments see the body's design as a reengineering challenge. As a result, we have persuaded ourselves that health and life are not connected to the way our hearts beat and lungs fill with air, to the way we stand on two feet and hold our heads high; nor to the way we extend a hand and bend our thumbs, walk and run, twist and turn. These are incidental considerations. There's always another way, a better way. That's what we tell ourselves.

Why, then, do such approaches so often provide no escape from chronic pain? I believe that being truly pain free depends on rediscovery, not reengineering. By rediscovering the body's design and allowing it to work as intended, many of the disabling conditions that take such a financial and personal toll can be reversed or avoided altogether. While we do need to grasp some basic anatomy, our starting point is common sense, based on practical experience. I promise I won't get too technical: First, though, we will have to spend a few pages reviewing why the body occasionally—more than occasionally, for some of us—uses pain for its own important purposes.

Chronic musculoskeletal pain is a form of high-priority communication. It warns of impending danger. "Something," pain seems to be announcing, "is happening that shouldn't be happening." Identifying that something is left to us, which is the problem. To put a stop to the pain, we go looking for what's wrong in order to correct it. But we don't have many obvious choices. The leading one is the muscles, which move the bones through the mediation of joints. These elements become the focus of treatment. The cure comes down to eliminating or managing this muscle-bone movement as

> **Pain is also telling us something is _not_ happening that should be happening.**

much as possible. After all, the pain goes away, doesn't it? As a matter of fact, it doesn't. Chronic pain is so designated precisely because it is intractable—it comes and goes and then comes again. The message it is sending us is really quite different from the one we think we're getting.

What is not happening is adequate motion. The big cosmic question, Why are we here?, will perplex humankind forever. But from a musculoskeletal standpoint, the answer shouts at us from our very first glance at the human body: We are here in order to move! The body is a motion machine. The bone-levers and the muscle-pulleys make that perfectly clear. They account for sixty percent of the body's weight. We may have a high purpose, but physical movement, hand over hand, one foot in front of the other, is how we accomplish it. Does it seem logical, therefore, that the body would ever send us a message that we must limit our motion or stop moving altogether? It is highly unlikely; if we move too much, simple fatigue is ample warning that we should rest. Why, after three million years, would we suddenly need to limit or manage muscle-bone movement?

Actually, we don't. But our extreme aversion to pain and our unwillingness to heed the body's other, less urgent messages have led us to make an all-out assault on the very mechanisms that protect our health and keep us pain free. If damaged joints, bones, and muscles appear to be the source of pain, then they are regarded as diseased. These structures may indeed show signs of wear and tear and abuse, but the conditions that cause the pain cannot be addressed by joint surgery, therapy, or other site-specific treatments. There is no artificial replacement for motion. Motion is absolutely crucial to the body's operations and overall welfare.

Motion as Both a Reaction and a Choice

Human beings are among the minority of living creatures that are not moved, at least on some occasions, by natural external forces. For us, there is no drifting with the tide, gliding on currents of air, or hitching a free ride on another organism. Either we move ourselves, or we perish. Consequently, the means and methods by which we move are as close to indestructible as nature can make them. The turtle got a hard shell to be able to hunker down and endure; we were given sinewy muscles, sturdy bones, and pliable joints in order to grow, to walk, to run, to move—and thereby to endure. Bones, however, do only what muscles tell them to do; and muscles take their orders, via nerves, from the brain. This chain of command allows us to take the first step toward achieving that higher purpose that I mentioned a few paragraphs earlier. What makes us human is not merely the fact that we can only move under our own volition. It is not even the fact that our brains respond to what is going on around us. With human beings, more than instinct is involved. We evaluate, deliberate, and choose. Our reactions to external stimuli keep the body fueled and capable of motion. The more we move, the more we are capable of moving.

From the instant the human fetus first kicks or shifts its position in the womb, it is moving in reaction to its environment, and it will continue to do so for the rest of its life as long as the environment provides one key ingredient—stimulus. The brain must be externally stimulated if it is to move skeletal muscle. But today the fetus eventually emerges into a modern environment that demands of it less and less motion. This lack of stimulus is affecting all of us, young and old. Today, unlike our ancestors, we may choose not to move. In modern life, moving appears to be optional. Thus, what we do to work and play no longer fully engages our major musculoskeletal functions. The biomechanical paradigm is reversed: The less we move, the less we are capable of moving.

Learning to Recognize Nonpain Symptoms

Pain has one and only one function: to alert us to danger. Chronic pain is not telling us that we are frail, or that our bodies have lost the ability to cope with the physical demands of life on earth. It is warning us of danger; and the danger is acute motion starvation. No longer do we sufficiently walk, run, or otherwise react to what was once a motion-intensive environment. Our systems are in a dysfunctional state—they are not being refueled by motion. I know this because, based on my work with clients at the clinic, I know that the body is using other forms of communication besides pain to tell us that dysfunction is happening. Even aside from pain, the body is letting us know that motion is in short supply. We get sluggish and stiff, and we start to hurt. Our knees and feet turn outward, our shoulders become rounded, or our hips become misaligned.

Helen, for example, came to the clinic from her home in Canada wondering why she had recently been losing her balance so frequently. She'd fall on the stairs at home or after getting up from a chair; the slightest stumble or sudden change in direction when she walked would result in an embarrassing crash landing. She hadn't had any major injuries, just bumps and bruises, but to be on the safe side, she wanted to find out what was going on. Was it an inner ear problem? Poor eyesight? Was she getting frail? As we talked, she told me that since retirement, her favorite activities were reading and going to the theater—both of them inactive pastimes.

> **DYSFUNCTION:**
> **A DEFINITION**
>
> I'll define dysfunction by providing an example. One of the neck's functions is to allow the head to turn to the right and left in a 180-degree arc. The inability to do that, and any other routine movement, is a dysfunction.

Having clocked up thousands of hours sitting down in the company of her favorite authors and actors, Helen's life had such a total lack of motion that the muscles she depended on for balance were no longer strong enough to do the job. She couldn't walk in a straight line and had taken to unconsciously hanging on to the walls or the furniture as she moved around. Plus, her back was hurting. But after the first hour in the clinic getting a motion "fill up"—deliberate stimulation of key posture and gait muscles—she was again walking in a straight line and was relieved of her back pain.

Just as a person with a fever may have a flushed complexion, the body openly displays symptoms of ill health and dysfunction. Once we see the problem on display, we may then correct it ourselves. Self-care is the earliest form of medical care—the doctor was not "in" three million years ago.

But we are ignoring these messages too often, obliterating them with stimulants, pain-killers, surgery, and ergonomic palliatives that try to make the body conform to man-made operating procedures and standards.

I was first confronted with pain symptoms as a twenty-two-year-old. After working summers as an agricultural laborer, playing varsity college football, and undergoing Marine combat training, I had gone from peak physical condition to a state of constant pain and disability, in the instant it took for a stranger to squeeze a trigger. There was no slow transition. After I was wounded, I became a different person; I could see it, feel it. I looked in the mirror and remembered how, a short time before, I had stood upright, walked, and done simple things like tie my shoes. Not only couldn't I do those things any longer in the same way, I didn't look the same as I attempted them. My body moved differently; the input and output of the motion itself had changed. That old motion-driven template, still vivid in my mind, was what I set out to restore during my rehabilitation. In due course, as I got closer and closer to the model and my functions returned, I learned that the body does have a standard design, and that deviation from it is the source of pain and incapacitation.

> **THE THREE "R'S"**
> **OF THE EGOSCUE**
> **METHOD**
>
> **Rediscover the body's design**
> **Restore function**
> **Return to health**

I've been sharing that lesson ever since, first with other injured Marines and then with people in pain who have come to my Egoscue Method clinic when they found that drugs and surgery were not the answer. For them, and for you, rediscovering the human template is the first step to becoming pain free.

The Shape of the Spine Makes Us Human

The obvious components of the musculoskeletal system are the muscles, joints, bones, and nerves. Within this assemblage are both hard and soft tissue and—in the case of cartilage, tendons, and ligaments—material that is both hard and soft, spongy yet resilient,

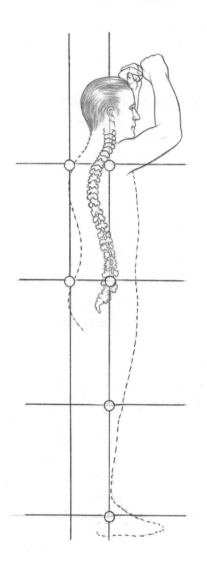

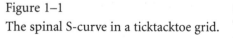

Figure 1–1

The spinal S-curve in a ticktacktoe grid.

flexible as well as rigid. If I stopped right here, I could be describing a fish or a bird or, for that matter, any vertebrate. What sets us apart from all other creatures grows out of the arrangement of our muscles, joints, bones, and nerves. Like our vertebrate cousins, human beings possess central spinal columns, yet we part company with the rest of the family (except the great apes) in that our spines are shaped like an elongated S; this allows us to stand erect on two feet and to take our spines with us when we move. The lovely S participates in bending forward and back, rotating laterally to the left and right, and wiggling, waddling, stretching, and dancing through myriad planes of motion.

The spine's S-curve is the centerpiece of a geometric construction based on parallel vertical and horizontal lines and ninety-degree angles. These lines intersect at eight joints—I call them load-bearing joints—of which there are four on each side of the body: the shoulders, hips, knees, and ankles. Try to visualize a skeleton enclosing a skeleton, which is what the horizontal and vertical lines amount to. The arms, rib cage, pelvic girdle, and legs are all suspended upon a perfectly balanced superstructure that, if turned sideways and viewed at a slight angle, with the S-curve in the center, resembles a three-dimensional ticktacktoe grid (with four horizontals instead of two) (figure 1–1). The ninety-degree angles are formed at the points of intersection.

Our stable skeleton's skeleton is precisely what a competent scaffold rigger would build. Anything else, and the whole thing would tip over and fall to the ground. Without parallel lines, hold on to your hard hat. The rigger uses clamps to fasten the structural pipes in place to hold the ninety-degree angles. The body does the same with ligaments, tough bands of tissue that attach bone to bone through the mediation of joints. But getting the structure to stand upright is only half the battle. Unlike the scaffold, the body must also move smoothly—forward and backward, obliquely and laterally, by crawling, walking, running, climbing, and leaping.

SMP: Standard Muscle Procedure

Here the muscles come into play, to move the bones. But they are not any old muscles and any old bones; rather, specific muscles are assigned to shift specific bones by contracting and relaxing. They perform this task within the skeletal design context of parallel lines and ninety-degree angles. And this musculoskeletal function, in turn, arises in association with stimuli from the environment. External stimuli are basically translated by the nervous system into internal responses. If, for example, I see a friend in the distance, I raise my hand to wave. There is a stimulus and response: Without seeing my friend, I wouldn't wave. If I were stranded alone on a desert island, I would not use the gesture. Eventually, both my memory of the gesture and the muscle to perform it would vanish.

> **Musculoskeletal functions are retained only through regular use.**

Use of the musculoskeletal system is thus linked to external stimulation. It is impossible to overestimate the importance of stimuli to the musculoskeletal system or, for that matter, to all the other systems. The nerves signal the muscles to move the bones only for a reason. One of the oldest reasons—and it is still as current as your last meal—is an empty stomach. When hungry prehistoric humans were engaged in the search for food, they had to walk uphill and down, run to escape predators, climb trees to pick fruit, and so on. The result was that they developed a set of working physical functions keyed to the demand for food—to the ongoing environmental stimulus. If a predator was in hot pursuit, they ran. If there were tempting fruit trees, they climbed.

> "We are what we eat," the old saying goes. Actually, we are what we *do* to eat.

If saber-toothed tiger was on the menu, the prehistoric humans would have to have functions ranging from cunning and stealth to speed and strength if they were to satisfy their hunger. From prehistoric times to about the twentieth century, the world was physically a very stimulating place for humankind. The earth was a terrestrial obstacle course, with wild animals, forest fires, towering mountains, bloodthirsty enemies, trackless deserts, and surging waters. Faced with these obstacles, our early ancestors developed thousands of biomechanical responses (biochemical, as well) keyed to environmental stimuli, then bequeathed them to later generations. Our musculoskeletal system today is the product of the unceasing influence of this environmental stimulation. We look the way we do—when we are fully functional—because our demanding environment literally sculpted our muscles and bones. It is our fate today to live in a modern world with ancient bodies. That's not to say the musculoskeletal system is frail or obsolete. On the contrary, it has withstood a torturous three-million-year road test.

I see the signs of musculoskeletal dysfunction all around me, in the form of converging and diverging—that is, nonparallel—lines. The skeleton within a skeleton is out of plumb. The scaffolding is sagging. Heads, shoulders, hips, knees, and ankles that are intended

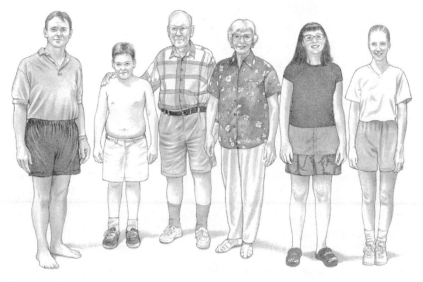

Figure 1–2
A group of people exhibiting "sagging" dysfunctional effects in different ways.

to interact and operate on the same planes are forward, rounded, rotated (and/or elevated left to right or right to left), laterally torqued, and everted (figure 1–2). Muscles and bones are fighting gravity, and gravity is winning. Meanwhile, the S-curve of the spine is being pushed, pulled, and compressed until it starts looking more like an I, an inverted J, or a C, without the lumbar, cervical, and thoracic curves. This distortion is the problem we look for in the Egoscue Method Clinic—and we find it *everywhere*.

A Disease Called Civilization

An estimated thirty-five million Americans suffer from some form of chronic musculoskeletal pain. Two out of three adults in the United States experience at least one major incident of back pain. And those figures don't take into account Europe, Asia, or the rest of the industrialized world, where the problem is probably just as severe. The human body is confirming how hyperadaptable it is.

To survive as a species, Homo sapiens successfully adapted physiologically to the world around them. What were conditions like when human beings developed? The question is still being debated by scientists, but one of my favorite bits of nonscientific evidence is a chunk of pure white marble. Michelangelo's famous sculpture of David in Florence is the artistic *embodiment* of thousands of years of motion. If the shape of the sculpted stone bears any resemblance to the real-life muscles that Michelangelo saw around him, it reveals what conditions were like in the vast expanse of time preceding the fifteenth century. David's harsh environment, and that of his ancestors, have fashioned his body into a machine capable of killing the giant Goliath. The figure looks almost godlike, yet still and all, it depicts a human being. In the shoulders, the sinuous back, the rugged hips, and the powerful thighs, a Renaissance genius captured the secret of our success as a species: We adapt. We grow strong, smart, and gloriously transcendent through motion.

Just as David's biceps are a reflection of the mechanism of adaptation to an environment that demanded a shepherd boy have the physical ability to hurl a stone with deadly force and accuracy or see his flock destroyed by predators, musculoskeletal dysfunctions are also a consequence of human adaptability to our own life circumstances. By not triggering latent biomechanical responses, our environment is literally deprogramming and crudely reprogramming the musculoskeletal system through the body's adaptive processes. As microbiologist and author René Dubos noted in his 1968 Pulitzer prize–winning book *So Human an Animal,* such processes are not always beneficial: "Evaluated over the entire life span, the . . . mechanisms through which adaptation is achieved often fail in the long run because they result in delayed pathological effects." Thirty years ago, Dubos was noticing this breakdown of the interplay between humankind and the natural forces that have shaped us. He concluded that many of the "diseases of civilization"—crime, violence, and stress, to name a few—are the result of responses to environmental factors. Humans seem to have adjusted to the modern environment, but, in fact, they are experiencing seriously detrimental consequences.

In the case of the musculoskeletal system, there are two stages to pass from a normal functional state to a pathological condition. First, the body shuts down organs it does not use. Why? In situations of scarcity—situations in which humankind found itself for millions of years—superfluity of any kind was a threat to survival, a drain on precious resources. Therefore, even today, muscles that are not being regularly stimulated are put on hold to atrophy until they are again needed. The second stage is purely adaptive. Every now and then, even the most sedentary man, woman, or child is asked to run, climb stairs, bend over, or pick up a heavy object. To perform such a task, involving the movement of bones by muscles, the body, aware that the assigned muscle is not capable, *borrows* another muscle to get the job done. Driven by the certain knowledge that it must move, it hijacks peripheral muscles to do the work that should be done by major postural muscles were they not atrophied. That is, the body improvises or adapts in order to survive.

Do you see how these three "-tion" words powerfully interact?

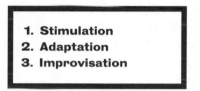

1. **Stimulation**
2. **Adaptation**
3. **Improvisation**

The body is pulled "out of joint," and it loses its parallel horizontal and vertical lines when borrowed, improvising muscles do the work of major muscles.

Peripheral muscles lack the power and design proficiency to do their own assignments *and* the work of the main posture muscles. Moreover, the peripheral muscles take a beating over time, and their own design functions become compromised. Dysfunction leads to more dysfunction. The body knows it has to move those bones somehow, so it goes farther and farther afield to find substitute muscles and ingenious combinations of what I call *compensating muscles.*

Many people who come to my clinic try to bend over at the waist using the muscles of their upper thoracic back and walk with their abdominal muscles. Darla was one of them. In the clinic, when we asked her to take a deep breath, the petite young woman's stomach hardly moved. Her abdominals were contracted, and when she walked, there was very little swing in her left arm. These are two important symptoms of dysfunction in the hips and upper back. Instead of performing their proper role as spinal stabilizers, lateral trunk and rotational muscles, and secondary posture muscles, the abdominals were being used to help position and swing the legs. Meanwhile, the muscles of the upper back were going into contraction to substitute their rigidity for the weak abdominals and hip muscles. When the foundation of a building gets shaky, the upper stories brace to provide stability. Darla had the classic restricted arm swing of someone with a bound-up thoracic back. You can spot it on the street as people walk or jog along—one arm will hardly swing at all. When they try to bend over, the upper back does most of the work; the dysfunctional hips and low back have a limited ability to swing forward and down. To compensate, Darla looked as if she were trying to fold herself about a third of the way down her trunk, as her knees flexed to help her bear the weight.

ARE COMPENSATING MUSCLES DIFFERENT FROM OTHER MUSCLES?

There's no physiological difference. The compensating muscle is one that has its own assignment but is being used for other purposes, even though it is unsuited for the task. Secondary and peripheral muscles are the usual candidates, as major primary muscles opt out from disuse.

Yes, it is possible to walk with your abdominals and bend over with your thoracic back. The body permits it, I believe, in emergencies or unusual situations. Important muscle groups may atrophy because of injury, illness, confinement, or other factors. But these conditions, given a varied, physically stimulating environment, are supposed to be temporary. Instead, the dysfunctions are lasting whole lifetimes—lifetimes of pain and incapacitation.

Understanding the Body's Bilateral Nature

These dysfunctions under the rigors of modern life are *not* a reflection of the body's inferior design. Nor are pain and dysfunction the price we must pay for growing older, being women, jogging, swinging a golf club, or holding certain jobs. On the contrary, the body is responding in strict accordance with the logic of its own musculoskeletal heritage. What's illogical is that we ignore the body's design as we go about our daily lives and submit to medical treatment.

When it comes to the musculoskeletal system, we're not the ones who make the rules. All the body's organs, its bones and muscles, are already governed by a coherent, comprehensive canon of rules. We can only understand and follow them. As basic as that may sound, it is a radical proposition in light of an attitude that presupposes that medical science can substitute its own notions of how the musculoskeletal system operates. We don't need a new and improved musculoskeletal system. The old one would work just fine, if we let it.

> **Bipeds are bilateral.**
> **(So are bicycles.)**
> **Why? Balance.**

The design of the human musculoskeletal system is universal. Rare birth defects and genetic anomalies do not even remotely account for the contemporary epidemic of chronic pain. For most people, saying "I was born this way" or "That's just the way I am" is the equivalent of saying "I was born without the need for oxygen" or "Gravity just doesn't apply to me." Only at our peril can we ignore our body's need for a full range of stimulus and response within a vertically and horizontally maintained parallel skeletal matrix. Equally perilous is our disregard for the body's symmetrical and unitary nature.

The eight load-bearing joints that I mentioned earlier are

MISALIGNMENT AND CHRONIC PAIN

An elevated right shoulder or a rotated left hip is dysfunctional for the simplest reason of all—the right shoulder is supposed to look and act like the left shoulder. They do identical jobs. The same goes for the hips, knees, and ankles. All the components work *together*—up and down, right to left.

arranged in four pairs, distributed on the left and the right sides of the body. Each side was created equal and alike in terms of upright load bearing, leg, shoulder, and arm articulations, and other functions. When the eight load-bearing joints don't all work together, "I was born that way" isn't the explanation. Rather, compensating muscles have moved those bones and joints out of their proper positions, and while they may not hurt, they are symptomatic of a dysfunction that is robbing the body of its ability to move according to its basic design. Moreover, the dysfunctional joint is affecting the integrity of the musculoskeletal system as a whole. Getting the body into an upright position and keeping it there is a major undertaking that engages the entire body, from head to toe. The badly worn heel of your right shoe (the left seems brand-new) may have as much to do with your stiff neck as with your aching feet. The condition of the shoe is as much a symptom as the pain itself.

That's good news. A worn heel is a lot easier to fix than a herniated disk in the spine. Instead of waiting for pain to drive us to seek treatment, we can take action before it starts to hurt. Conventional pain-abatement procedures have not addressed the problems that continue to undermine health. This book is filled with good news. The best of it is that the body's design gives you rights—the right stuff and a birthright—to be pain free.

THE BODY'S DESIGN: A FIRST-CLASS MECHANISM BATTERED BY SECOND-CLASS TREATMENT

You are about to read a horror story. It is one of the few in this book; most of the other stories are case histories about people who were able to reclaim their birthright to be pain free. Alex wasn't so lucky. But what happened to him is the proverbial picture that's worth a thousand words. Instead of spending several pages explaining why the convergence of two historical developments is seriously endangering our health, I'll tell you about a man whose wrist hurt.

A Cure Worse Than the Disease

Alex is in his early fifties. After a successful career in professional football, he retired to spend time with his family and start a business. While he was still playing football, Alex would occasionally come into the clinic for minor injuries and conditioning work. I hadn't seen him for a few years, and when his name appeared again on my appointments schedule one day, I figured it was more for a social visit than anything serious. When he walked into the office, he was carrying a large envelope under one arm.

"I know you, buddy, you're here to sell me something," I said, joking, knowing that he is as fiercely competitive a businessperson as he was as a football player.

Alex shook his head. "No, I'm not selling anything." He dropped the envelope on my desk. I noticed that his right wrist was heavily bandaged and braced. "Would you mind taking a look at this?" He sat down in front of the desk. "I want to see what your reaction is."

X-rays. I held the first sheet up to the light. Huh? I closed my eyes in disbelief and snapped them open again to get a better, wider focus. My jaw dropped open. "Where's the radius? A good two inches are gone!"

Alex nodded and told me what had happened. He had been having some wrist stiffness and pain, although nothing major. One day, early the previous December, he had been golfing. The round had been going well, until a sand trap got in the way. As he swung the sand wedge to get out, an excruciating pain in his right wrist dropped him to the ground. He went to see his doctor immediately. After an assortment of tests, he was told that the radius, the smaller of the two bones of the forearm that run from the elbow to the wrist, was damaged. He would need to have an operation to correct it.

"My doctor said they'd go in and clean things up," Alex related. "I remember he added that in the worst case—which wouldn't happen—they might have to shave some of the bone." When he woke up after the operation, Alex said, "I knew something was really wrong." When the doctor arrived, he explained to Alex that the bone was just too far gone and that a substantial piece had had to be cut out.

I took another look at the X-ray. The radius terminated roughly two inches above the point where it should have converged with the ulna. Any tendons that were in the way had simply been reattached elsewhere. The truncated radius, which moves in close relationship to the ulna, was lashed to its partner with borrowed ligaments to keep it from wandering around. The two condyles of the ulna and radius (the knobby ends of the bones) form half the wrist joint; the other half is composed of eight independent carpal bones in the arch of the hand-wrist, held together by a complicated intertwining of ligaments. Removing the radius's condyle eliminated about a third of the wrist joint's mass, leaving its outer edge totally and permanently unstable. It was anybody's guess what the effect on the carpal bones would be. Yet it was through this carpal obstacle course that the tendons had to thread in order to supply the thumb and fingers with muscle power. Would they hold their positions? Would the reattached tendons change the way muscle contraction and relaxation was handled?

"What was the disease?" I asked. There had been no sign of malignancy, and no follow-up treatment along those lines.

Alex shrugged. "Bone disease," he said, with more than a bit of bewilderment tinged with sarcasm. He wasn't laughing, but he knew crying wasn't going to bring the bone back.

Then I saw the "disease." It was in Alex's shoulder. Rounded forward and down, his right shoulder had repositioned his elbow, which was interfering with the wrist function. The radius was probably taking a beating. Realigning the shoulder would have relieved the pain and eliminated the stress on the bone.

I put Alex on an E-cise therapy program that almost immediately eliminated the swelling and pain from the operation. Over time I believe that he will recover much of his wrist function, but it will take a lot of work; otherwise his wrist will serve primarily as a decorative device for attaching the hand to the forearm.

The episode is an example of high-tech pain-killing at its worst. The surgeons had used a technique on Alex that had been developed for extreme forms of traumatic joint and bone injury, the kind of accidents that crush musculoskeletal structures. Alex had been hitting a golf ball, not holding his wrist under a steamroller. That his doctor would treat someone for a single incident of acute wrist pain by reengineering the joint, the way you'd slap together a quick repair on a faulty conveyor belt or crane, shows that we've become so intoxicated by modern tools and techniques that we are casually sacrificing the body's most indestructible and vital mechanisms. Once experimental and highly risky, invasive medical technology has become relatively commonplace because of a reflexive demand for maximum treatment; a piling-on of procedures that only a few years ago would have been used with great reluctance and only in worst-case situations. Like a military arms race that has run amok, bigger and bigger guns are being rolled out to fight smaller and smaller skirmishes.

Coupled with our abundance of conveniences and an absent-minded redefinition of health that has established pain control as the overriding consideration, this inappropriate use of technology has created a crisis that is threatening to turn one of the strongest species of vertebrate life into one of the weakest and most endangered. The human body—Alex's and yours—is under siege, and it is slowly losing its viability.

Pain in Perspective

Think of pain as the body's own built-in car alarm. Tamper with the knee, shoulder, wrist, whatever, and the howling starts. It's an effective method, really, for protecting these joints and their associated muscles and nerves from further damage. The pain is not only a *grabber,* it is a *stopper.* It tells us to knock it off and fix what's wrong—now!

But where a car alarm brings the owner running to protect his or her precious vehicle, modern medicine has learned how to silence the warning shouted by pain. The thief, however, is still at work. What's being stolen, in the case of the musculoskeletal system, is strength, mobility, dexterity, confidence, and joy.

But since the slow theft doesn't hurt, who cares? And besides, nobody ever dies of knee pain, right? Wrong. Death comes, although it is slower. The *bad* knee takes its time, but it immobilizes the individual and sets in motion a sequence of profound physiological occurrences that are then blamed on age, gender, genes, or disease. The climax isn't immediate or obviously linked to an instantaneous cause, so the sole object of treatment becomes the elimination of pain in the knee. The inevitable consequence that the function of the joint will be impeded—and it surely will be—

or that the person will be incapacitated or die, are remote events that will not occur for months or years, so they are not regarded as relevant to the treatment.

This attitude comes in large part from misconstruing joints as simple, or at least as less complicated than the major internal organs. Rather than biochemical, joints are biomechanical in nature. Many of the components of the musculoskeletal system resemble simple and familiar hinges, or balls and sockets, or levers and pulleys. Therefore, tinkering with them seems like no big deal. The neighborhood Volvo mechanic does it all the time. It makes perfect sense—or it would if your body had been made on an assembly line in Sweden.

Since it wasn't, we have to stop treating the musculoskeletal system like a second-class anatomical citizen.

The design configuration of each joint and its associated musculature have their own logic and purpose. Modern medical science, as slick as it is, simply isn't slick enough to successfully impose a twenty-first-century design on a circa 3.2-million-year-old musculoskeletal system. Nonetheless, the deceptively simple appearance of the shoulders, hips, knees, and ankles tempts intelligent men and

---

THE STARTING LINE

Confronted with the command to run, the body seeks extra oxygen. This is what follows next: Anchored in the lower part of the chest cavity under the lungs, the diaphragm muscle contracts and moves downward to decrease pressure in the chest, thereby drawing air into the lungs—the bellows; then, as the dome-shaped diaphragm relaxes and returns to its original position, carbon dioxide is expelled; twenty to forty liters of it for the average person per hour. Meanwhile, in conjunction with the dropping pressure in the chest cavity and a change in blood chemistry (extra carbonic acid molecules) triggered by muscle function, the heart—the pump—kicks over at an increased heartbeat rate to quickly circulate freshly oxygenated blood to nourish the hardworking muscles.

women to try to fix what isn't broken. If some function suffers along the way, it's a small price to pay for being without pain. This misguided attitude, if applied to the heart or liver, wouldn't last long—nor would the patient. Yet with the musculoskeletal system, it is assumed that the function—walking, stretching, twisting, turning, or bending—is of secondary importance in terms of overall health, and that it can be relatively easily jury-rigged to work almost like the real thing.

> **The joints are as complicated and as simple as a kidney.**

Almost isn't good enough. There's too much at stake. On the most simplistic level, the musculoskeletal system operates both as a bellows and as a pump. This similarity is most obvious when we run. For the initial stride, the nearly unconscious act of extending the anterior—swinging—leg is more than an isolated muscular accomplishment, restricted to the hip, knee, and foot. Dozens of muscles, perhaps hundreds, both striated and smooth, are engaged by the biomechanical and biochemical performance.

Try it yourself: Take a few quick strides. Immediately your lungs will begin to fill with air. What do thighs have to do with lungs? Everything, when it comes to the action of our bellows and pump.

> **Every system of the body is energized by motion.**

This sequence starts with a stimulus—whatever it was that prompted you to run—and continues with a long series of interrelated responses, ranging from adjustments in the twitch rate of major muscle groups and cartilage thickness in the joints, to variations in skin temperature and glandular activity. That is, the stimulus initiates motion, without which the entire sequence falters. Motion is involved, therefore, even in the operation of bodily systems that are not direct participants in the rough-and-ready business of getting from point A to point B. The involvement of the body in taking a single stride is total.

By misconstruing the musculoskeletal system as exclusively involved with posture and locomotion, we have failed to appreciate its central respiratory, circulatory, and metabolic roles. Thus, when a middle-aged man says, "I don't walk much anymore because my knees hurt," we regard the statement as meaning only that he will have to cut down on his caloric intake to avoid gaining weight. What's happening, though, is that his systems are beginning to shut down, which impedes and weakens his internal systems and organs. His complaints will slowly escalate from "I can't walk because of my knees," to "I've lost my appetite," "My stomach hurts," "I can't sleep at night," "I feel dizzy," "I have high blood pressure," and so on. These are all effects of motion starvation.

> ### ROTATION
>
> **Most joints operate like levers or hinges; they open and close, moving two bones together or apart. Meanwhile, rotation also occurs. The joint's components move internally—up and down, side to side, forward and back—to allow for growth and flexibility. But if rotation becomes the primary moving force in the joint, there will be damage.**

Inner and Outer Health Are Closely Related

Kevin is a real estate attorney who has spent most of his life sitting down: first in a schoolroom, then at a desk in an office, in bucket seats in cars, and in an easy chair in front of the TV. His major muscles assigned to the task of walking are no longer capable of doing so with the required efficiency and effectiveness. For the most part, unused hour after hour, those muscles have been shut

DO MUSCLES SHORTEN AS THEY LOSE DESIGN MEMORY?

Muscles always remain the same total length. While their fibers contract and relax, muscles do not stretch or shrink. With dysfunction, gradually less and less muscle fiber is involved in a muscle's work. This usually starts in the extreme ends of the muscle and works toward the middle, making it seem like the muscle is shortening.

down, and the body has redirected its resources elsewhere.

However, he occasionally needs to go to the bathroom and visit the cafeteria for lunch. In other words, Kevin must walk at least a little bit. These brief walks, though, aren't enough to maintain the musculoskeletal functions that are needed even to reach these nearby destinations. He ends up borrowing peripheral muscles and bypassing the quadriceps, the major muscle group on the front of the thighs. Normally the quads would stabilize the knee, guarantee its ninety-degree angle of operation, and position the hip. Without the quads, however, extra rotation is introduced to the knee joint, and lateral stress pulls it out of alignment with the hip and ankle. Given this situation, it is inevitable that Kevin will one day encounter sore knees. He'll blame it on the jogging he used to do, but the real cause will be lack of motion. As he travels farther down this long road, his dizzy spells will make the motion-health linkage even more vivid. Not only did his lifetime of sitting interfere with his ability to walk, it also undercut his capacity to breathe. Major posture muscles are not the only ones that atrophy from disuse. All muscles—actually, all living tissue—share that characteristic.

Without sufficient stimulus from his environment to demand motion of Kevin, his diaphragm—that dome-shaped shelf of muscle under the lungs—gradually forfeits its full range of motion and capability. As he moves less and less, reducing his physical activities, his diaphragm loses its *design memory*. Its powerful contraction and relaxation decrease simply because Kevin isn't using much of that function. In time, it hardly moves at all. As for his quads, their flabbiness grows in direct proportion to the flabbiness of his diaphragm. Other muscles in the torso—among them, those that primarily function to move the arms, head, and spine—take over the diaphragm's job of getting oxygen into the lungs, without being nearly as competent.

As a result of the reduced oxygen, Kevin's brain, which uses about forty percent of the total oxygen intake of the body, begins to starve. It does not do so without a long struggle: Paramount as it is, the brain diverts oxygen to itself from less essential functions, running the gamut from locomotion and posture to digestion to the production of white blood cells and beyond. Meanwhile, chronic pain makes itself felt. Joints and muscles that lack oxygen cannot function properly, no matter how they are drugged, manipulated, or surgically altered. All the other systems suffer as well.

Health in Twenty Minutes

How much motion is enough? The amount, measured by the time spent performing design movement, varies from person to person, relative to the degree of total anatomical functionality. Usually, it pertains to what the individual does for a living and the other physical activities he or she normally pursues. Surprisingly, time-wise, it is not very much, thanks to the body's great efficiency. For a functional person whose lifestyle is moderately active, as little as twenty minutes a day spent deliberately providing sufficient motion requirements is enough to maintain musculoskeletal health. Those who are totally sedentary—mega–couch potatoes—would need an hour or more, but that's entirely hypothetical since someone in that state has no chance of becoming

---

THE ROUTE TO PROPER MOTION

The E-cises in the upcoming chapters will work on restoring proper design motion to the joint that's afflicted with chronic pain. The overall conditioning program in chapter 13 is geared to the whole body.

functional without a change in lifestyle that includes at least moderate levels of physical activity.

The upside of beginning an exercise program is that as musculoskeletal function returns, the person's desire to be more active steadily increases. In the clinic we have to watch our clients closely to make sure they don't try to go too far too fast, propelled by the joy, confidence, and energy they experience from even a modest reawakening of long-slumbering functions. Three months of short daily workouts stabilize most badly dysfunctional musculoskeletal structures enough to allow for a shift to a gradually more physically active lifestyle.

As for *proper* motion—design motion—what you see is what you've got. It's either there or it isn't. If it isn't, that's conclusive evidence of insufficient and/or improper motion (usually both). And I should add that indiscriminate movement is never a substitute for sufficient and proper movement. There is no such thing as functionally sufficient movement that is not proper movement as well. To be absolutely clear: By *proper movement,* I mean design motion that is in keeping with the vertical, horizontal, and parallel alignment of the eight load-bearing musculoskeletal joints. In addition, the head rides atop the S-curve of the spine, on the same axis as the shoulders, hips, knees, and ankles.

Without proper design motion, we are looking—whether it is in your mirror or the therapy rooms of my clinic—at the posture of chronic pain.

Law and Order

One of the education missions that we perform at my clinic is to teach people that neither bodybuilding nor grinding workouts can replace or activate lost functions. All the stair-climbing in the world would be a dead loss for Kevin, whose disengaged, unused quads will be inaccessible to him until he persuades the lower half of his powerful adductor muscles to butt out of the walking process. The StairMaster (and the treadmill and the stationary bike) would actually be strengthening his adductors and increasing his dysfunctions, not to mention severely torquing his misaligned knees.

WHAT'S AN ADDUCTOR?

Adductor muscles draw a body part toward the median plane of the body. The hips, for instance, have powerful adductors that allow us to draw our thighs, knees, and ankles together. Abductors perform the opposite function.

We can move it and still lose it.

There is motion and there is design motion. Only design motion restores health. Motion that is at odds with the design is, at best, wasted; at worst, it is harmful. It is possible to systematically restore functions that will result in proper movement and in the maintenance of a fully functional musculoskeletal system—and in being pain free. Kevin and many people like him don't understand that the body is neither mysterious nor hideously complicated. It has hard and fast requirements, but none that we can't easily comprehend. Actually, its operating principles can be summed up in eight points.

The eight laws of physical health constitute a checklist that we can all use as we shop the megamall that the health care system has become. We can compare the products that we're being sold—be it a prescription drug or a surgical procedure—with what we really need. When one or more of the eight laws doesn't square with the effects of the product, something is wrong. Hip replacement surgery is an example of a product (and a profitable product as well, for hospitals, surgeons, and physical therapists); does it violate the law of vertical loading? Absolutely! I have never seen an individual who has undergone the procedure who wasn't seriously out of vertical alignment, both before and afterward. It's the rea-

THE EIGHT LAWS OF PHYSICAL HEALTH

1. **VERTICAL LOADING**: Gravity is necessary for health. In order for gravity to exert a positive and dynamic influence on the body, the skeleton must be vertically aligned in its postures.
2. **DYNAMIC TENSION**: A state of constant tension exists between the front of the body and the back. The posterior portion is responsible for the erection of the body and the anterior is responsible for the flexion, or bending forward, of the body. Neither activity can be performed correctly and healthily without this action.
3. **FORM AND FUNCTION**: Bones do what muscles tell them to do. All skeletal motion is initiated by muscular activity.
4. **BREATHING**: The body will not function without oxygen. So essential is this law that the body has redundant systems to ensure compliance.
5. **MOTION**: All of the body's systems—digestive, circulatory, immune, and so on—are interrelated. The common thread that binds them together is movement. The faster the molecules of the body move, the higher the metabolic rate. The higher the metabolic rate, the healthier the human being. We are designed to run, jump, climb, fall, roll, and skip, not just for initial development but for continued health throughout our lives. If these activities hurt or cause pain, it is because we are violating some or all of the laws of health.
6. **BALANCE**: In order for the law of motion to be effective and true, the body must achieve balance, defined as muscle memory, sufficient to constantly return the body to the first law of vertical load. For balance to occur, muscles must work in pairs *and* equally on the right and left sides of the body. Being left- or right-handed hinders this balance only when we violate the laws of motion.
7. **STIMULUS**: The body reacts to all stimuli twenty-four hours a day, regardless of the conscious state of health. Therefore, the law of motion constantly reinforces this law of stimulus. If motion is limited, the law of stimulus becomes stressful to the body. The body absorbs pollutants and irritants rather than deflecting them.
8. **RENEWAL**: The body is organic; therefore, it is in a constant state of growth or rebirth. Muscles, bones, nerves, connective tissues, cartilage, and the like are all alive. If the body is not renewing, it is because we are violating the laws of physical health. The more laws we violate, the faster we age and die.

son for most hip pain and why most hip replacements fail, but I'll go into that in detail in chapter 7. In the meantime, it's enough to say that much of what we are being sold doesn't even come close to conforming to the eight laws.

And that's why you're not pain free. It's why, as author and reader, you and I are engaged in this dialogue. Being pain free is possible; you've already taken a major step in attaining it by reading this far. Going the rest of the way, though, must be done on a strictly do-it-yourself basis. Now that you're aware of the body's design and its operating principles, I'll show you how the Egoscue Method pulls all the elements together to help you do it yourself. Then it will be your turn.

3

THE EGOSCUE METHOD: GETTING PERSONAL TO STOP CHRONIC PAIN

If I ever go into the bumper-sticker business, this will be my first one:

> **Bones do what muscles tell them to do.**

It's a message that needs the widest possible exposure. You may have noticed that this is the third time it's appeared in this book. Don't be surprised if you see those words again, on several more occasions. I hope you'll get so sick of them that you'll ask in exasperation, "Okay, what do the muscles say?"

Good question, I'm glad you asked. The answer provides the fastest, most direct avenue to being pain free.

The Body Has Its Own Weather Channel

A recent magazine article about the alternative health technique known as biofeedback summarized a key concept as "getting in touch with your pain." Really? It seems to me that for most people who are hurting, their number-one priority is to get out of touch with their pain as fast as possible. There is validity, though, in the concept of getting in touch with your body. We tend not to be aware of our physiological systems beyond the most superficial level, things like being uncomfortably hot or cold, suffering from a bloated feeling after overstuffing ourselves on pizza, or feeling an urgent need to empty the bladder or the bowels. Likewise, we usually fail to tune in to the effects of a gradual deterioration of our musculoskeletal and other physical functions. Small losses accumulate over time without overtly registering on us. Sensitive to a receding hairline, an emerging paunch, or a new crop of skin blemishes—living on the surface—we are numb to the workings of the inner body. But numbness is not a sign of good health.

MUSCLE MEMORY

Much of the success of the Egoscue Method is based on its ability to reconnect individuals to their innate kinesthetic sense, or muscle memory, of how things feel beneath the surface. It is more basic than remembering that an overstuffed suitcase is going to be heavy or that a long walk in loose shoes will lead to blisters. Kinesthetic sense allows us to respond physically to the experiences that we have archived in our long-term memory. Suppose my mind needs to know if my muscles and other physiological systems are capable of getting me up eight flights of stairs in a hurry. It reads the musculoskeletal system much the way a pilot checks his instrument panel before he decides to pull back on the stick and lift off. This internal assessment is taking place constantly, and the output not only results in a decision to hit the stairs or wait for the elevator, it leads to the creation of a general operational climate of health.

Each of us lives within his or her own health "ecosystem," acting or reacting consciously or unconsciously to the weather prevailing there. When a group of people wait to crowd onto an elevator when it would be faster and less hassle to take a few stairs, the reason is not laziness or bad habits. Rather, the kinesthetic sense is announcing to each one of those people, "Forget the stairs—the demand required cannot be comfortably or safely met by existing functions." And it is also conveying important information about stress levels, anxiety, and fatigue. The pilot checks the gauges and aborts the takeoff.

Kinesthetic sense works in the background, which is why there is often a disconnect between it and our consciousness. We see in-your-face foreground events—nagging kids, traffic, an unreasonable boss—as the reasons we are having a bad day. But our kinesthetic sense knows that we are having a bad year or bad decade due to gradually declining functional capacity. Over time, the climate turns bleak and inhospitable. Without realizing it, we no longer associate wellness and well-being with using our bodies the way they were intended to be used. Physical activity stops feeling good to us. When we lose that elemental reference point, we lose our bearings. We don't know what makes us feel healthy, and worse, we don't know what makes us feel sick.

When this numbness finally gives way to pain, muscle memories demand our attention. When the pain persists, the conclusion is "I have a case of chronic pain" that needs drugs, surgery, or some other radical treatment. Pain, however, is only one of many muscle memories. A key premise of the Method is that it is possible to both feel and see painless muscle memories—symptoms—of musculoskeletal health. Once that happens, once the kinesthetic sense is back in business, an accurate *personal* assessment can be made of what needs to be done—and what doesn't. Pain is no longer driving the process.

The word *personal* is set in italics in the preceding paragraph for a good reason: The Method recognizes that musculoskeletal health does not depend on intermediaries. It is, to use a term favored by MBAs and other business types, a form of disintermediation: There's no middleman. You are put back in charge of your own muscles and bones. You don't have to be an orthopedic specialist, yet *feeling, seeing,* and *understanding* the basics of this biomechanical process are essential. Ignorance may be bliss for most of us when it comes to the mysteries of auto repair, computers, or lawn care, but for our musculoskeletal systems, ignorance is pain.

Unfortunately, it's not at all unusual for clients to come to the Egoscue Method Clinic whose only reference point to their bodies is pain. Their attention is riveted to the spot that hurts; all other sensations are blotted out. As functions are restored, the pain abates. But once the clients become aware of these restored normal musculoskeletal operations, a new disorientation and even panic set in. Worried, they report a new problem—"I've got this pain in the back side of my thigh." What is happening is that they are feeling their hamstrings for the first time in years; but all they know is that something unfamiliar is happening. They have no objective standard as to what a functional ankle, knee, or hip feels like. And the reverse is also true: They have no objective standard for what dysfunctional joints or muscles feel like—until they start to hurt.

The Method supplies that missing standard—nothing less than the body's own design—and allows the individual to see it (often for the first time) and feel it. After a long spell of amnesia, recovering those muscle memories is exhilarating and empowering. I probably sound like a broken record during a typical day in the clinic as I ask people who are doing the E-ciscs, "What's that feel like?" The responses start out as "I don't know" and evolve into "Funny," "Better," "Stronger," "I can feel it in my knee now," "My shoulder seems looser," and so on. Throughout the process, I'm also asking the person to look at her body in order to reinforce the fact that what she is seeing, she is also feeling.

Over the years, I have found that people absorb information in different ways. All of us use three tools—sight, sound, and touch. Even so, the degree to which we employ them varies from individual to individual. Some people learn faster by observing a demonstration; others understand more quickly if they listen to an explanation; still others need hands-on experience, learning by trial and error. The Method uses all three approaches. It starts with the head, by providing a basic grounding in the way the musculoskeletal system operates; Biomechanics 101 without pop quizzes or final exams, as in the first three chapters of this book. The next step is to develop the capacity to perceive the mechanisms at work in oneself and others—seeing is believing. Finally, it comes down to mastering the ability to be cognizant of these functions as they actually take place.

I admit that my goals are ambitious: I want to change the way you think, see, and feel. All three goals are essential.

Nobody else can move those muscles—and muscles that don't move lose strength and function. On this point there are no exceptions. The musculoskeletal system was designed to maintain itself in a motion-rich environment, and does not readily take to management by drugs, surgery, or other forms of outside therapeutic intervention. All that's required is motion in keeping with design requirements and an adherence to the integrity of that design. The experts, no matter how well trained and well-meaning, can't do that. They add or subtract to the basic equation—motion + design = function—and the outcome is subtly or drastically altered. Most "cures" are ultimately based on limiting motion; however, all this does is compound the problem by further weakening the muscles and guaranteeing that even that limited amount of motion will eventually be too much to bear, and pain returns. The most well-meaning advice, "Stay off it," "Wear a brace," "Take these pills three times a day," "Fuse the spine" offers disruption instead of repair, when all it takes is to follow the instructions the body gives us with each step we take.

> **Just as you cannot delegate eating, drinking, or sleeping, you cannot pass the buck when it comes to operating and maintaining your own musculoskeletal system. It is strictly a self-service mechanism.**

Changing Basic Definitions: Jane's Story

Modern medicine is driven by pathology, which is the study of abnormality. Consequently, the gateway to health is through the back door, past disease and illness. This approach has steeped physicians and scientists in what's wrong with the musculoskeletal system (and all other systems and subsystems) rather than what's right with it. Understandably, dysfunctional individuals seek medical treatment more than functional individuals do. There is no problem as long as everyone understands that dysfunctional cases are, in fact, abnormal.

In the last thirty to forty years, however, as our society has become more sedentary and the incidence of chronic joint pain has escalated dramatically, the criteria of normality and abnormality have been whittled away until only outright disfigurement (one vivid example is osteoporosis), acute immobility, and pain are considered abnormal. A host of other symptoms of musculoskeletal dysfunction—stiffness, fatigue, poor balance, rounded shoulders, loss of the spine's lumbar curve, obesity, and many other conditions—are regarded as normal.

One day a client of mine from Washington, D.C., stepped on a glossy magazine that skidded out from under her and fell, breaking her right ankle in six places. Jane asked her doctor if the incident was unusual, and he said, "No, not at all. People go out to their front steps for the newspaper, trip, and bingo—it's very common." He didn't say a word about her *valgus stress,* a common dysfunctional condition of the knee in which hip displacement causes the knee joint to twist laterally toward the inside of the leg, so that the descending weight torques the ankle down and under along the inside edge of the foot (figure 3–1).

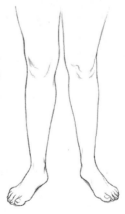

Thus, while the accident was precipitated by stepping on the magazine, the cause of the injury was valgus stress. A functional hip, knee, and ankle would have allowed Jane to recover her balance or, at worst, to take a minor tumble. But thanks to thousands of accumulated hours spent sitting down, Jane's adductor and rotational muscles have taken over from the main posture and gait muscles (the ones that flex and extend the hips, knees, and legs). When she walks,

Figure 3–1
Knees with valgus stress.

that right knee visibly tracks to the inside and the foot flips out, pivoting on the heel, and rolls inward—if it's on a stable surface. She's "normal" as long as she has no pain and doesn't encounter a glossy magazine (and so are several million other people with the same easily correctable condition).

Perversely, the abnormal has become normal. The ankle, a rugged utility vehicle that makes the Land Rover seem like a kiddie car, breaks in six places when an otherwise healthy woman stands up to answer the telephone in her own comfortable office. Nobody asks, "What's going on?" because, to quote her doctor again, "It happens constantly."

As more and more people present injuries related to musculoskeletal disorders, it is increasingly assumed that the dysfunctional state is the state of nature: that different people with different lifestyles all have different inadequate designs. The frightening thing is that this conclusion is accurate. The body adapts itself so well to an increasingly motionless environment that it superficially redesigns itself to cope with the lack of stimulus. The trouble is that the redesigns—not the design—are inadequate in the long run. This redesign phenomenon is becoming so pervasive that we are losing the functional musculoskeletal template. Even when we see it, we have increasing difficulty recognizing it. Medical research, for example, is being routinely conducted these days with subjects who, because they are not reporting symptoms of pain, are regarded as having healthy, *normal* musculoskeletal systems. This seriously undermines the results of the research: Obviously, if you are conducting a double-blind study on, say, whether a particular physical activity is beneficial in preventing back pain, you are likely to arrive at a false conclusion.

A study done in 1996 at Stanford Medical Center concluded that forty percent of people over forty years of age have degenerative or bulging spinal disks, even without developing disabling symptoms or serious disease. The conclusion was that such disks are a normal part of the aging process, akin to a few gray hairs. Sorry, bulging disks are not normal at any age. They are a symptom of a musculoskeletal disorder, a pathological condition that compromises the spine's ability to flex, rotate, and bear weight. Something's wrong here. Only Orwellian doublespeak turns sickness into health. That's why it's such an urgent task to change the way we see the musculoskeletal system. We must relearn the oldest way of perceiving our bodies: Pain or no pain, if it looks sick—wobbly, weak, drooping, twisted, off balance, limping, bent, stiff, or frozen—it is sick.

Changing Perspectives Through Technology

The musculoskeletal system's worst enemy, though there are a number of runners-up for the distinction, is the X-ray machine. With one stroke of technological genius, we went from observing the body from the outside with two sharp eyes to scrutinizing it with a specialized instrument from the inside.

I'm not a complete Luddite. X-rays do answer many important questions. But they do so at a high price. For one thing, we no longer trust our eyes. The outward appearance of the musculoskeletal system has come to seem irrelevant. What we end up looking at, furthermore, is the site where there is pain and visible damage, because we mistakenly believe that the problem lies there. Without the X-ray, as for most of human history, the health care provider and the patient would be forced to concentrate on the outside of the body, where they would make an accurate diagnosis based on what they saw with their own eyes. An elevated shoulder, a rotated hip, a misaligned knee, and other visible distortions of the musculoskeletal system provide valuable information that is now mostly overlooked because technology directs our attention elsewhere. Instead of observing those obvious surface anomalies, asking why they exist, and acting to correct them, we are distracted by beguiling pictures of pathological conditions that are not of primary significance.

Seeing is believing, yet if what we are seeing merely reflects what technology is able to frame, what we believe to be true may well be flat-out wrong. From that point on, things go awry. Based on misimpressions created by sophisticated technology, procedures are devised using more sophisticated technology to address causes that are, in fact, effects. The cartilage loss in a knee or calcium buildup in the spinal canal are spotted by the hardware, and means are created to take care of those specific situations. In the end, the patient gets a new knee or a carefully widened spinal canal. But the real biomechanical cause is unaddressed, so it continues to put stress on the new knee and deposit calcium in the new spinal canal. This effect won't show up in an X-ray until months or years later; in the meantime, the individual has apparently been cured of his or her pathological condition. In reality, all that has happened is the suppression of one set of symptoms, one muscle memory—pain. If the other symptoms are still present, then illness remains.

Having condemned this obsession with pathology, I have to acknowledge that the Egoscue Method is also concerned with pathological conditions and that it uses technology as well. Our equivalent of the X-ray is the snapshot, taken by a small digital camera. Until recently we used a thirty-dollar Polaroid, but we've since gone digital in order to load the images into our computer system. Basically, we take four pictures of the client: a frontal view, from head to toe; a rear view; and two side views. Each picture also shows a decidedly low-tech carpenter's plumb line. With these simple images, the client is able to see easily that he or she lacks vertical and horizontal alignment. Like a scaffolding that is beginning to collapse, the musculoskeletal system has lost its ninety-degree angles, and that is a serious pathological condition.

If the patient brought along a set of X-rays, I might say, "The X-rays show cartilage loss in the right knee. Do you think that might have something to do with your elevated right shoulder? Here, take a look at the snapshot."

Silence.

"Do you see where your hip is?"

"It's elevated, too."

"How about your feet?"

It doesn't take long. People start seeing that one half of their body is doing something decidedly different from the other half.

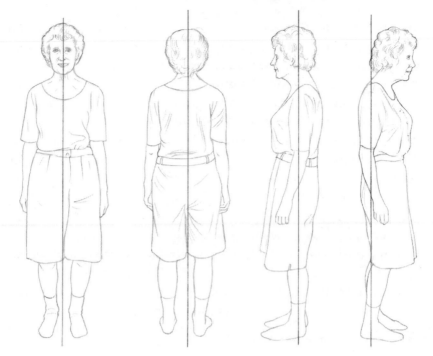

Figure 3–2
A nonbilateral body.

E-cises: The Unworkout That Works

And the cure for this dysfunction? Motion. The Egoscue Method fills the stimulus gap created by the sedentary modern environment with a unique program of exercises targeted at muscles and functions that are receiving inadequate or improper motion. One of the additional reasons we call them E-cises (beyond the Egoscue-cise label that I mentioned in the introduction) is that they have nothing to do with the traditional kind of strengthening or bodybuilding exercises that people usually associate with hard workouts at the gym. E-cises amount to muscle and joint *tutorials*. If motion deprivation establishes itself, our bodies literally forget how to move according to design. E-cises reteach the muscles what to do and how to do it.

Participating in E-cise tutorials is similar to sending your dog to obedience school. Suppose Rex is a good watchdog but has a bad habit of ripping apart shoes when he's left alone. Obedience school will retrain him to do his job as protector without devouring your best loafers. Egoscue Method tutorials are designed to return compensating and substituting muscles—those that are performing nondesign functions—to their design roles.

Keep in mind that compensating muscles are active muscles; as such, they tend to be stronger than the inactive muscles that are supposed to be performing a specific musculoskeletal function. Therapy that ignores the imbalance between active and inactive muscles will fail because the stronger active muscles will keep their predominance. To show you how this works, let's go back to Jane, whom I mentioned earlier, with her fractured ankle and valgus stress. After her cast was removed, her physician advised her to do an exercise to promote flexion and extension of her right foot. The technique he recommended uses the lower leg as a lever to operate the ankle hinge joint forward and back. It was a good idea. Nevertheless, after doing the exercise for some time, Jane's right hip and knee were still out of place, held there by strong muscles. When she tried to lever the right lower leg forward, it twisted inward to the left. As conscientiously as she tried, it was impossible for her to restore normal foot flexion and extension until her hip and knee were neutralized and restored to their design position. If that didn't happen, and Jane kept at it, she would actually be building the strength of compensating muscles and thereby reinforcing her dysfunction.

FLEXION-EXTENSION

Flexion takes place when the muscles draw two bones toward each other. If you clench your hand into a fist, that is an example of flexion. Extension moves bones away from each other. These are extremely important functions. If either one is lost or impaired, there are serious consequences.

Our two-tiered approach gave Jane an E-cise program that worked on her hip dysfunction first. Then, as that dysfunction backed off, other E-cises gradually transferred proper knee function and foot flexion-extension back to the correct muscles. As this transfer was happening, Jane could see and feel her hip, knee, and ankle repositioning themselves.

How Muscles Can Regain Strength and Balance

The Egoscue Method is unique in recognizing that therapy programs succeed only when they treat the body as a closely integrated unit. Ignore the three factors in the accompanying box, and you're headed for failure.

All the long muscles in our bodies form unbroken chains, via the joints and long bones, that stretch from head to foot. They also interact closely with short, localized muscles. Many common strengthening exercises, pieces of gym equipment, and therapeutic routines attempt to isolate certain muscles or muscle groups. Two favorites are the abdominals and the quadriceps. The idea is to focus the workout for quick results. But muscles never operate alone and when they return from temporary and artificial isolation there are consequences up and down (and across) the entire body. Fortunately, we don't have to do that. Muscles know their place and have their own work to do; they will readily return to their proper function with a moderate amount of encouragement. As they do, they and the compensating muscles will resume their balance and strengthen themselves equally as components of the overall unit.

> 1. The work of a weak, inactive muscle is being done by another muscle (or muscles).
> 2. Strengthening a weak muscle isn't enough, because compensating muscles are likely to absorb the entire stimulus, leaving the weak primary muscle unchanged and at a greater disadvantage.
> 3. Efforts to isolate muscles do not work as intended since muscles always function in close cooperation and collaboration with other muscles.

Many of the E-cises in the following chapters are variations on familiar exercises drawn from yoga and other disciplines. Techniques for manipulating the biomechanical component of the human body have been around for centuries, mostly as means to enhance endurance, speed, and balance. Still, no ancient yoga master, Renaissance fencing instructor, or Victorian-era proponent of wooden Indian clubs and leather medicine balls ever anticipated a time when motion would become scarce.

How to strengthen your quads or abs is no mystery. The real challenge is to strengthen them in an environment that provides inadequate stimulus to the parts of the body that work *with* those quads and abs.

A REMINDER ABOUT THE E-CISES AHEAD

The E-cises in the chapters that follow are meant to stop chronic pain by restoring design motion to your body. They will usually do this within twenty minutes of beginning the E-cise menu. I recommend doing the E-cises in the morning so you benefit from them all day. At a minimum, you should experience a significant reduction in pain by the end of your first session. So don't be discouraged if some of the pain lingers temporarily: Give it twenty-four hours, then repeat the menu. You will make progress. Resist the temptation to speed the process by increasing the number of repetitions of individual E-cises. At first, your body will be able to usefully absorb the effects of only limited amounts of stimulus; I have factored this into the instructions. And don't try to take any shortcuts! Where called for, do the E-cises for both sides of the body, even if the pain is only on one side. When the pain abates, keep doing the menu daily for at least two weeks, unless otherwise instructed. You are the best judge: When you feel pain free, go to the overall conditioning program in chapter 13. Do that menu daily to ensure that the pain will not return. If you miss a day, don't worry—just resume the routine. But if a long interval goes by, return to the original menu for a few days in case the layoff created instability in the musculoskeletal structure. Soon the E-cises will be making you feel so good that you'll rarely miss a day.

FEET: THE CARE OF THE SOLE

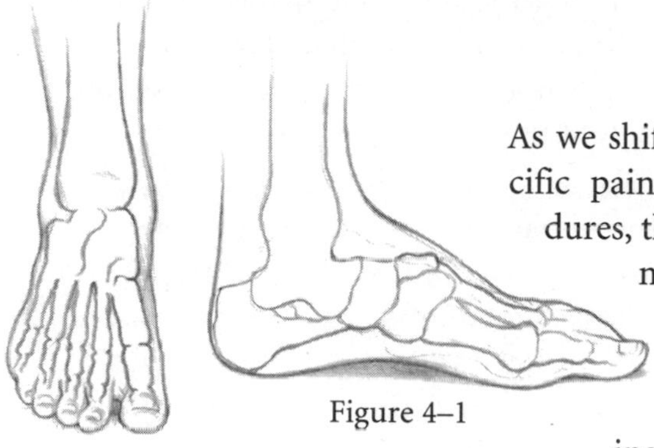

Figure 4–1

As we shift the focus to specific pain treatment procedures, the head would be a more elegant starting point than the feet. But practically speaking, the feet are where the means of locomotion unique to humans—upright movement—begins. Our fully erect posture, a feature we share with no other creature, rests on two feet.

Little Feet, Big Job

We have a love-hate relationship with our feet. We alternately abuse and pamper them, ignore and fuss over them with everything from pedicures to Air Jordans. No other body part generates anything close to the billions of dollars we spend to keep our feet comfortable, sexy, and hip. At the same time that we are treating them like royalty, we expect these same feet to toil like peasants, and never complain. When our hardworking feet do break their code of silence with pain, we subject them to another huge industry dedicated to gagging their cries for help with moleskin, orthotics, massages, surgery, and a host of other measures.

Even though they may seem puny, the feet are not fragile. What they lack in bulk and surface area, they make up for with an ingenious design based on two simple arches, one longitudinal and the other transverse. The tarsal and plantar arches use the bones of the feet, including the toes, to form medial and lateral beams (figure 4–1). Arches, as any *archi*tect can tell you, have tremendous strength and flexibility. The arches of the foot support the entire weight of the body and simultaneously allow it to stay upright as it moves across varied terrain, balancing the load as it shifts. To do this smoothly, the arches have to retain their shape, and the foot must strike the surface of the earth in a way that allows the arches to flex and otherwise function properly. Most foot pain is a symptom of an absence of one or both of these prerequisites.

Fallen arches, or flat feet, became a running joke during the Second World War, when military doctors started granting 4-F status to draft-age men because of the condition. But flat feet are nothing to laugh about. As a Marine combat officer in Vietnam, the last thing I wanted to do was train or fight with troops that had flat feet. Why? Because they have poor endurance, they are accident-prone because of impeded balance, they are slow to get out of harm's way, and they have difficulty carrying heavy loads. And they have two more liabilities as well: Their feet get tired easily and hurt much of the time.

When the foot loses its arch, the sole, comprised of short muscles, small bones, tendons, and ligaments, comes in direct contact with the ground (figure 4–2). The foot has no shock-absorbing capacity without the arch, which means that as the dysfunctional foot strikes the ground, it sends the impact waves right up the bones of the lower leg to the knee and beyond. That's just for starters. The bones, muscles, and nerves of the sole also form an intricate mechanism for transmitting data to the central nervous system. Just as the fingers and palms of our hands are able to evaluate a surface to determine whether it's rough or smooth, hot or cold, healthy arches react in subtle and minute ways to changes in the terrain beneath them. The soles send

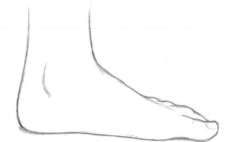

Figure 4–2 A flat foot.

that information out to the brain for processing. The brain orders the muscles in the lower leg to flex and extend, in order to position the ankle joint for the next step. Meanwhile, the foot itself, distributing the body's weight evenly from heel to toe, goes on to accomplish a small liftoff maneuver and prepares for the next touchdown.

In a foot with fallen arches, the muscles of the sole stay in perma- nent contraction. As happens when we clench our hands into fists, much of the sense of touch is lost. When the muscles of the sole are "clenched," they can make little or no differentiation in their response to the terrain. Deprived of a functional sole, the muscles of the calf, knee, hip, and low back must take over the jobs of orchestrating load distribution, carrying out the foot strike, and performing surface evaluation and response. Unsuited to footwork, however, these mus- cles and joints sacrifice the nuances of essential foot function to the crude necessity of keeping the body on its feet and moving forward.

In the process, two perfectly useful and essential functions— supination and pronation—are compromised and corrupted. Both terms need to be explained. The foot flexes and extends not only from heel to toe, but also from side to side. Pronation, which you've proba- bly read about in magazine articles on athletic shoes, is the mechanism by which the inner edges of the feet react to the terrain when we take a step while walking, or to impact when we jump. The foot rotates in- ward, and the foot lands on its inner edge. Supination is similar but in- volves the outer edges of the feet, when we push off to jump or lift the foot to walk. Pronation and supination are paired muscular functions.

The pronator and supinator muscles accomplish these move-

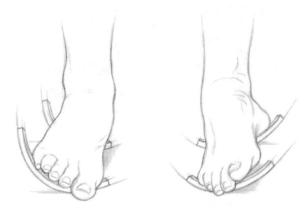

Figure 4–3
A foot on cradle rockers, showing pronation and supination movements.

ments. It is as though the foot were sitting in a cradle, rocking from side to side (figure 4–3). But without supination and pronation, the feet clomp along, striking the ground rigidly, devoid of lateral adjustments and, without that motion, unable to accommodate variations in the terrain. Their supination and pronation functions are taken over by other load-bearing joints. The powerful lower leg and hip muscles improvise an emergency technique to maintain a semblance of balance: They evert the foot, turning the toes outward and the heels inward. This adjustment achieves a small measure of lateral flexibility and balance, but it sacrifices the heel-toe gait pattern of weight distribution and articulation. The other joints, too, stop operating according to design.

> **Muscles always pull—they can't push. One moves a bone to point B, while another moves it back to the starting place at point A.**

Pronation is improvised, providing more stopgap foot flexibility and balance, when the individual develops a new way of taking a step: by pushing off with the inside edges of the feet, like a skater. The muscles of the hip that were normally involved in pronation are now used for step-by-step movement, but they are not set up to flex and extend the foot properly. All they know how to do is operate the inside edge of the foot, which becomes bladelike.

In this dysfunctional state, the foot and ankle are extremely unstable. As a result, the joints above—the knees, hips, and shoulders—no longer have a firm platform. To move the body forward without toppling over, these joints start using extra rotation, which makes for extra wear and tear—and pain. During this dysfunctional pronation, the knees and hips rotate inward, increasing the downward pronating pressure on the transverse arch of the foot. That contributes to the fallen or (as I prefer) failing arch. The weight of the body is being focused on the inside edge of the arch, rather than distributed evenly. It's like the roof of a house that has several tons of snow piled on just one end. The arch goes from overburdened, to sagging, to collapsed (figure 4–4).

Meanwhile, in dysfunctional supination, the foot moves up and twists out along the opposite outer edge. But it is unable to get into position to receive a solid impact on the bony heel and the fleshy ridge across the ball of the foot; therefore, the structure of the foot is literally pounded into the ground. The same process happens even when the arches are intact but weak and semifunctional, compromised by knee and hip dysfunctions.

This is exactly what happened to Charles, whose arches had "started to go," he said, when he was a teenager. I met the World War II veteran after he had been through surgery on his left foot. The doctors had told him that his arches were "completely shot" and that the entire structure of his foot was in jeopardy. This sounded reasonable to Charles, who had been kicked out of the navy in 1941 and been refused enlistment in the army because of acute flat feet. Over the years, he had used inserts and special shoes, but in his seventies he finally underwent surgery.

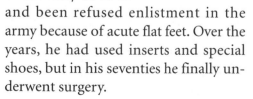

Figure 4–4
Flat, everted feet; the arrows illustrate the downward pronation pressure on the inside of the foot.

His recovery had been painful: He had done weeks of post-op physical therapy. Even so, when he came to the clinic, he was still limping and using a cane. Worse, his right foot was now hurting, and so was his back. I wish I could print Charles's comments about the prospect of another round of surgery. The language is too strong. Let's just say, he wasn't interested.

By using E-cises to work on his hip and knee dysfunctions, we were able to send Charles home at the end of his first session without his right foot and back hurting. He still had a lot more work to do, but getting the hips, knees, and ankles into better alignment—not perfect, just a little better—caused the pain symptoms to abate immediately. The arches in his right foot were allowed to bear weight and absorb impact front to back and side to side for the first time in about sixty years. And they could still do it.

A healthy foot strike—heel-toe, heel-toe, heel-toe—bears the impact across a surface area of eight or ten inches long by four or five inches wide (depending on the size of the individual foot). A foot that is everting (toes turning out like a duck) and supinating may lose two-thirds or more of this surface area, along with the all-important assistance of the knee and hip and their associated musculature. The pronating foot also has a drastic reordering of foot strike and loading capability, which you can replicate simply by standing pigeon-toed in your stocking feet for a moment.

Try it. Your weight immediately shifts into the inside edges of the feet, your knees stiffen, and your sense of wanting to topple forward increases. Also, if your hips are out of alignment and no longer

---

FLAT FEET

Flat feet are traditionally blamed on activities that require the person to stand in one place for prolonged periods. I believe that's incorrect and that the causes are actually musculoskeletal dysfunction, principally hip dysfunction. Shoes are also a factor when they hold the sole rigidly and deprive it of the ability to read the surfaces with which it is in contact and adjust itself accordingly. Held fast by the stiff sole of the shoe, the muscles of the foot atrophy.

bilateral (they probably are), you may notice that the vertical load is unevenly distributed between the two sides of the body. It will feel as though your foot and knee on one side are being pressed down harder than on the other side.

Short Term Versus Long Term

The musculoskeletal system works as a unit, and if one of the components fails, the others also suffer. This chain reaction of dysfunction complicates treatment. So where does treatment start?

The answer: everywhere.

I'm not kidding. The temporary mitigation of pain is relatively easy, so first take care of the pain in your feet. But then move on to address the ultimate cause of the problem by aligning your individual load-bearing joints. Do this by performing the exercise routines recommended for the ankles, knees, hips, and shoulders (see chapters 5, 6, 7, and 9). Don't forget, however, that getting rid of the pain is just the first step.

The immediate problem in all foot pain is improper foot strike. In other words, whatever the ultimate cause of the problem may be, the most noticeable symptom is a dysfunction in the way the foot contacts the ground, dissipates the impact, and bears and distributes weight. This foot pain can be eliminated because, as I argue, failing arches are not a permanent condition. The bones and muscles of the foot are no different from the bones and muscles of any other part of the body, and the same rules apply to all of them equally. If a stimulus—improper foot strike, in this case—is altered, the body will respond. If the musculoskeletal dysfunction that is disrupting proper foot strike and load-bearing is corrected, the arches will resume their proper role. It won't happen overnight, but it will happen. The feet have undergone years of pounding, yet their resilience is nonetheless waiting to be reclaimed with only a little effort.

Don't look for a different E-cise to treat each foot condition. The E-cises that start on page 53 address underlying dysfunctions that manifest in a variety of symptoms. Heel spurs, for example, can be treated the same way as bunions. How is this possible? Because the structures involved are the same, and all of them have the same problem. The only difference is the symptom itself—and you and I are treating the cause and not the effect of musculoskeletal pain.

Plantar Fasciitis and Heel Spurs

The plantar fascia is a tough sheet of connective tissue that attaches to the rear of the heel. It stretches fanlike under the sole and toes of the feet to form a lining of sorts between the skin and muscles. Plantar fasciitis is a condition that feels like one is stepping on a nail each time the foot hits the ground.

> ### FOOT STRIKE
>
> Any pattern of foot strike that deviates from heel-ball-toe is a symptom of dysfunction in the load-bearing joints. The structures of the foot are not designed to handle alternatives. Special shoes or inserts may make the feet seem more comfortable, but they do nothing about the continued stress in the ankles, knees, and hips.

The pain occurs when the fascia is inflamed, usually from friction caused by improper loading and foot strike. Frequently, this condition gets blamed on worn shoes or poor running technique, but both of these usual suspects are guiltless. The friction will be present even with brand-new shoes and even if the runner learns to stop slapping his or her feet down too hard. Orthotics, specially made inserts that are put inside shoes to change the way weight and impact are managed, can temporarily silence fascia pain by shifting the friction to another spot. But even after it moves, the problem starts at square one and quietly builds.

Heel spurs are painful tiny calcium deposits that are formed at the spot where friction is irritating the bone. A form of callus, they serve to protect the bone from stress and chafing. They are also often present when the fascia is inflamed. Removing the calcium deposit is the standard medical procedure, but doing so without removing the cause of the irritation (also standard medical procedure) means that the inflammation and the pain will eventually return. The body will continue to activate this protective mechanism until the *source* of the friction is eliminated.

Calluses and Corns

Like heel spurs, calluses and corns form small, tough pads of semi-hardened skin as a result of irritation and intermittent friction. In origin, they are all close cousins, if not siblings. Calluses tend to be bulkier and show up on the heel, the ball of the foot, or the big toe, where major recurring friction takes place. Calluses are formed almost as if the skin were being armored for protection against the relentless rubbing. Corns can be both hard and soft in texture; they appear between toes and above and alongside joints that undergo a lot of abrasion against shoes.

As a result, many people who have calluses and corns blame them on their shoes or on jobs that make them walk too much. But this assumption is wrong. It is reinforced, to be sure, when they stay off their feet and the problem seems to get better. All that's happening, however, is that artificially limiting overall motion is reducing the friction created by muscular dysfunction in the foot, knee, and hip. Suppose a letter carrier, who bears most of her weight on the inside edge of the right heel, develops a callus. She gets a transfer to work behind the counter at the post office. The callus is still forming, only more slowly, keeping pace with the reduced level of activity. Of course, the lack of motion will at the same time aggravate the primary dysfunctional condition—in her case, a hip misalignment—to the point that more and more friction will be generated by less and less movement.

Bunions and Hammertoes

A bunion is a calcification of the first joint of a toe. This ongoing process often hits the big toe hardest, although the other toes can also be affected. Here again the body is reacting to improper foot strike and loading: It restricts the mobility of the stressed joint by creating a swollen red cushion of bursal fluid at the friction point. In time, the cushion solidifies into a virtual rock, and the toe starts curving outward.

> The site of the pain is rarely the site of the problem.

Bunion removal is a common procedure. But what's also common and predictable is that the bunion grows right back in. One client came to my clinic in desperation after having had her bunions removed six times. After about four forty-minute sessions with us and the short maintenance program that's included in this chapter, she was rid of them forever. She did the program every day for three months and changed the dysfunction that was causing the bunions.

The same strategy works for hammertoes. These are toes that crimp downward in a desperate effort to provide shock absorption, balance, and traction to the foot. It's as if the toes, acting on a primordial instinct, are trying to keep from falling over by reawakening the lost dexterity of their ancestral primate cousins and gripping the earth's surface. Actually, hammertoes are trying to do work that in a functional foot would be performed by the arches, ankles, lower legs, knees, and hips. In the clinic, many clients are surprised when we begin to work on their hammertoes with hip E-cises.

Four E-cises to Counteract
Dysfunctional Loading of the Foot

> **Total time: Fifteen minutes.**
> **Times a day: Once in the morning.**
> **Duration: Do exercises daily until pain abates for twenty-four hours. Once the pain is gone, continue with the menu for one week before switching to the overall conditioning program in chapter 13. For nonpain symptoms such as bunions, use this E-cise menu for three weeks, and then switch.**

- Foot Circles and Point Flexes
  (Figure 4–5)

This E-cise restores ankle flexibility and strengthens the flexion and extension muscles. For Foot Circles, lie on your back with one leg extended flat on the floor and the other bent toward the chest. Clasp your hands behind the bent knee while you circle the foot clockwise thirty times. Meanwhile, keep the other foot on the floor with the toes pointed straight toward the ceiling. Reverse the direction of the circling foot and repeat. Change

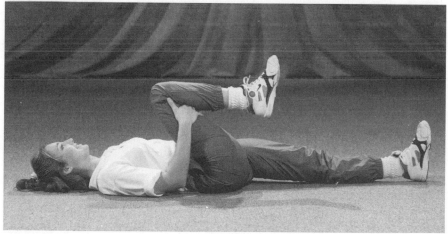

Figure 4–5

sides and repeat. Make sure the knee stays absolutely still, with the movement coming from the ankle and not from the knee.

　　For Point Flexes, stay in the same position on your back with one leg extended and the other bent. Bring the toes back toward the shin to flex, then reverse the direction to point the foot. Switch legs and repeat twenty times.

- SUPINE CALF/HAMSTRING STRETCH WITH A STRAP
  (Figure 4–6 a and b)

Lie on your back, with knees bent and feet flat on the floor about hip-width apart. For the Calf Stretch (figure 4–6a), use a belt or

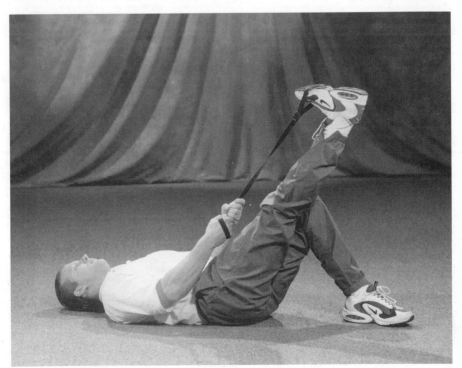

Figure 4–6a

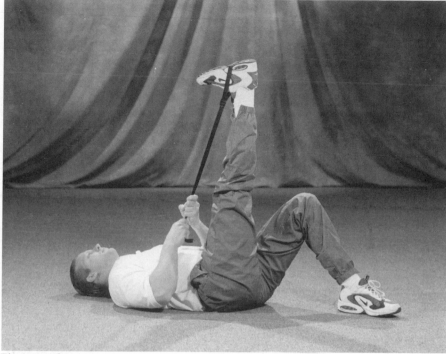

Figure 4–6b

strap with a loop in it to encircle the ball of the foot. Tighten your thigh while pulling the toes back with the strap. Keeping the leg straight, hoist it to about a forty-five-degree angle. The thighs of the straight and bent legs should be even. Relax your shoulders. Hold for thirty seconds. Repeat on the other side.

For the Hamstring Stretch (figure 4–6b), use the same position, but the strap should encircle the arch of the foot. Pull the entire leg toward your body, keeping it straight and the thigh tight. Be sure not to pull the leg too far (that is, do not allow the buttocks to lift off the floor). Hold for thirty seconds. This E-cise reintegrates all the muscles from the hip to the foot.

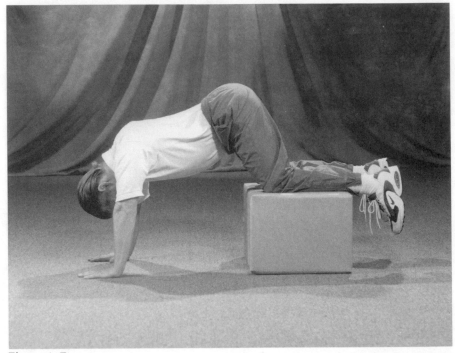

Figure 4–7

- STATIC EXTENSION
  (Figure 4–7)

This E-cise tackles hip rotation. Hips that not only rotate but actually twist to the right or left disrupt knee and ankle function.

Kneel on a block or chair with hands on the floor under the shoulders. Let your back and head relax toward the floor and shoulder blades come together. Relax. There should be a pronounced arch in your back. Keep your elbows straight, and shift your hips forward six to eight inches so that they are not aligned with the knees. Hold for one to two minutes.

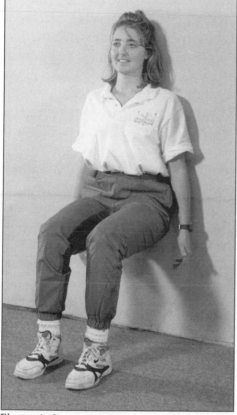

Figure 4–8

• Air Bench
(Figure 4–8)

This E-cise puts the hips, knees, and ankles simultaneously into extension while they are aligned and under load. The best way to get into this position is to stand with your back to the wall. Press your hips and the small of your back into it while walking the feet forward and simultaneously sliding down into a sitting position. Stop when you've reached roughly a ninety-degree angle. The knees should be over the ankles, not the toes. *(You shouldn't be able to see the toes.)* If you feel pain in the kneecaps, raise your body up the wall to relieve the pressure. Press the low back and midback against the wall to feel the quadriceps working along the top of the thigh. Hold for one to three minutes. This E-cise can be a bit of a struggle, but you do not have to be ultrafit to do it. If you feel like it is too much of a workout, then try it for only a few seconds and build up to one minute. Walk around for a minute after this E-cise.

Before I close this chapter, I need to address the issue of footwear. Pain or no pain, the rule here is classic: Less is more. From the standpoint of musculoskeletal function, the enemy of the human foot is the inhuman shoe. Encasing the foot in leather, canvas, rubber, or a synthetic fabric interferes with its function. The shoe's artificial sole robs the foot of its ability to flex and extend fully and to read the terrain beneath. The best thing you can do for your feet is to get them out of their shoes whenever feasible. Do as much walking as possible in your bare feet.

Pick shoes that are light, loose (not pinching or constricting), and flexible. The issue of heels is controversial. For women with a musculoskeletal dysfunction, high heels are a good-looking bad idea. They have a long list of negatives. For starters, they retard flexion of the foot and ankle, and they throw the weight of the body forward onto the front half or third of the foot. Some of their other sins include putting the calf muscles into contraction, freezing the hip and knee in extension, and encouraging the hips to roll forward and down to maintain an upright posture. Even so, all of that would be tolerable in an individual whose hips were functionally flat and square, but that's the exceptional person these days. All women, even functional women, are unstable structurally when wearing high heels. All have trouble changing direction in high heels because the heels so disrupt the normal gait-pattern that smooth muscular and joint interaction is impossible. On the functional woman, high heels will have no lasting ill effects, but it is one more blast of stimulus that the dysfunctional woman's body could do without. Still, if you absolutely must wear high heels, please don't blame your foot pain on the shoes. The cause will be a musculoskeletal dysfunction. Take care of that, and you can wear high-heeled snowshoes.

The same "less is more" formula goes for athletic footwear. Many manufacturers are using engineering and state-of-the-art technology to create shoes that accommodate their customers' dysfunctional feet, ankles, knees, and hips. But with every step they take in their engineered shoes, their dysfunction grows worse. They come to rely on their shoes for balancing, walking, running, jumping, and turning. In the process, the healthy musculoskeletal functions recede ever farther into the background. No shoes, no matter what the price or the brand, will cure foot problems. At best (and worst), they camouflage the dysfunction. A hidden problem only gets worse over time.

Shoes are an even more important issue for children. Adults may lose functions, and that's bad enough, but what's lost can be found. Children who wear improper shoes may never develop key functions in the first place. Indoors, children should be out of their shoes altogether. Whenever it's reasonable and safe, the same goes for outdoors. A summer spent barefoot in the park, on the beach, or in a back lawn will pay dividends over a lifetime.

The early months and years are crucial for awakening and strengthening musculoskeletal functions. The best place for baby shoes is therefore hanging on the car's rearview mirror—not on an infant's feet. Rushing to encase a baby's foot, even if he or she is walking, is a mistake. For one thing, as the infant wiggles, flops, and crawls, the foot is flexing and extending and growing in association with the muscles of the lower torso. Second, the shoe, acting as a platform, invites the baby to pull him- or herself upright. Although parents love to see their tots standing up, young children are designed to be quadrupeds for a reason. By rolling around, stretching, and contorting on their knees, hands, and elbows, they build total function from the ground up.

> **FOOT FAULT**
>
> Try this simple experiment: Take off your athletic shoes immediately after a workout. How does it feel to walk around? Turn quickly, stand on your tiptoes, walk backwards. Do you feel off balance? Less stable? If so, your musculoskeletal functions are telling you that they've grown dependent on the shoe and need them for support.

Forget timetables. Shoes are in order only when the child's gait-pattern is reasonably stable. At birth, his or her feet are rotated outward; they will start turning inward and straight ahead surprisingly quickly. By getting little Becky and Brent up on those everted feet too soon, then compounding the error with a pair of cute hard-soled shoes, they are being cheated out of their birthright. Don't be in a hurry. In due course, when everything is ready, the human body defies gravity and hoists itself upright to spend a lifetime on two feet.

5

ANKLES: THE CIRCUIT BREAKER

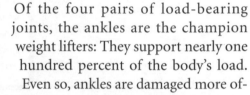

Of the four pairs of load-bearing joints, the ankles are the champion weight lifters: They support nearly one hundred percent of the body's load. Even so, ankles are damaged more often in athletic activities than any other musculoskeletal component, with the exception of the knees.

Figure 5–1

About twenty percent of all sports injuries involve the ankle. Games that require leaping, landing, making sudden changes of direction, and traversing rough ground account for most ankle damage.

Account for? Shouldn't I say "cause"? No: Basketball, tennis, volleyball, and cross-country running and walking are *not* to blame for ankle damage. Ankles can handle the requirements of an NBA playoff or a stroll in the woods with equal ease. A functional ankle can, that is. It's the dysfunctional ankles that get hurt while bird-watching or slam-dunking.

The Ankle—Weak or Strong?

Over many years as an exercise therapist, I've heard my clients use the expression "weak ankles" thousands of times. They use it to explain everything from why white guys can't jump to why intermediate downhill skiers can't cut smooth and linked turns. The ankle, according to this view, as the body's next-to-last connection to terra firma, is a relic of our past as quadrupeds; its very inadequacy proves that we were not intended to walk upright.

Nonsense. The ankle is a perfectly evolved mechanism for bipedal motion, in all of its variations and demands. By using the attributes of a hinge and a lever, it is capable of doing three things at once: bearing weight, moving weight, and managing high impact. The ankle, seen in X-rays, looks like a crazy jigsaw puzzle of skeletal components strapped together by rubber bands (ligaments), but the various articulations amount to a surface area totaling sixty percent of the entire unit. Instead of the cumbersome rigidity that would come from a few principal structural components, this gives the joint the capability of making nuanced, flexible, and resilient responses.

So why all the ankle injuries? Well, the answer actually is weak ankles. Unraveling this problem is the key to understanding the ankle. When the ankle is deprived of functional interaction with the knee, hip, and shoulder joints, as is the case when the load-bearing joints are misaligned, it is indeed weak. That abundant surface area—all the pieces of the jigsaw puzzle—becomes a liability instead of an asset. The ankle has too much play and responsiveness; the ligaments start snapping. Still, it's not the fault of the ankle. Like all the other load-bearing joints, it is in itself weak and insubstantial when it is in an *unloaded* state. All the joints need gravity and alignment to act as glue and give them strength. Fortunately, in a living human being it is impossible to unload the joints completely; if nothing else, gravity is still a factor. That means that the ankle always has some measure of strength. Not enough, though.

Ideally, the load-bearing joints achieve full strength when they all are engaged together as a single unit, much like a well-made dining-room chair. With its four sturdy legs, the chair will support guests for many years. But if people thoughtlessly tip it back onto its two rear legs often enough, it may start wobbling and ultimately collapse altogether. Similarly, left to themselves, the body's load-bearing joints lose the benefit of their combined strength when they do

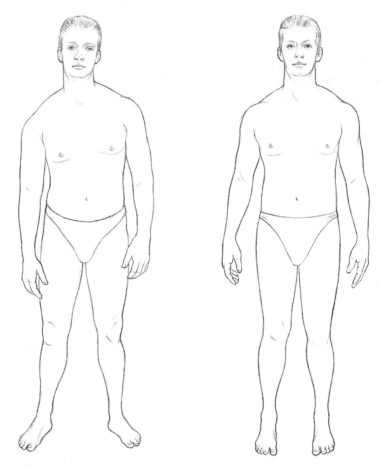

Figure 5–2
The body's load-bearing joints, dysfunctionally loaded and functionally loaded.

not function together. If the musculoskeletal horizontal and parallel lines (described in chapter 1) are lost, this vital combined joint interaction is compromised. The load isn't distributed evenly among the eight joints; the pressure bears down on some of them in isolation. It only stands to reason that as this occurs, the ankle, bearing as much weight and impact as it does, gets hurt often. But the solution is not a redesign of the ankle, splints, or special high-top shoes. A little help from its friends, the other load-bearing joints, will do the trick (figure 5–2).

Marc, a top NBA player, made this discovery when he came to

the clinic to have his knees "fixed." Since basketball is a sport where knee braces and bandages are macho badges of serious players, he regarded his knee injuries as an occupational hazard. We explained to him that the reason his knees were hurting was that his hips and ankles were disconnected. Their "wiring" was still in place, but they weren't communicating or working together much anymore.

Marc wasn't convinced, however, until he was asked to do the E-cise we call Foot Circles and Point Flexes (chapter 4, figure 4–5, page 53). Basically, it involves lying on your back with one leg flat and the other in the air. The upraised leg is bent at a ninety-degree angle and supported by both hands clasped in back of the knee. First the foot makes circles, clockwise and counterclockwise; then the toes flex and point forward and back. This E-cise is not difficult unless you have a dysfunctional ankle. Marc had almost zero range of motion in one of his ankles—an ankle on which he spent hundreds of hours jumping and landing, twisting and turning, and stopping and going as he played pro ball.

Of course, his knees hurt, and in time, so would his hips. When he realized the problem, Marc conceded that, yes, he had had his ankle scoped several times for bone spurs. (Arthroscopic surgery uses an instrument that allows the doctor to examine and work on the interior of the joint.) While he was matter-of-fact about it, spurs don't just happen. They are the result of grinding and pounding the ankle's components in isolation from the other load-bearing joints. The amazing thing (and even though we do this every day at the clinic, we are still pleasantly surprised each time) was that by doing the Supine Groin Stretch on Towels E-cise (chapter 6, figure 6–8, page 92), Marc went from zero to about eighty percent range of motion in forty-five minutes. The rest returned after a few more sessions—and his knees stopped hurting.

Ankle Sprains, Dislocations, and Swelling

All the various bony pieces of the ankle joint are held together by ligaments. These tough and relatively elastic bands of tissue can take a lot of punishment. It's been estimated that when we walk, the

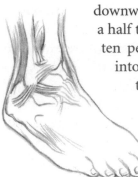

Figure 5–3

The ankle's fibular ligaments.

downward force on our ankles amounts to three and a half times our total body weight. At the same time, ten percent of the body's weight gets transmitted into the ankle as horizontal force generated by the inertia of forward movement. For a two-hundred-pound man, that's as if a twenty-pound bowling ball were rolling through the ankles, mostly front to back (if he's functional; if he's dysfunctional, the motion is side-to-side and from all points of the compass).

Because of such impacts, the ankle is designed to have a circuit-breaker mechanism; if it is overloaded with pressure (while unsupported by the other load-bearing joints), it will almost literally *blow a fuse.* The ligaments will be severely stressed: They will strain, tear in minor and major ways, and rupture, all in the interest of protecting the bones from fracturing.

The fibular ligaments, which attach the fibula bone of the lower leg to the ankle (one runs back toward the heel, the other forward), are the most frequently damaged structures of the body (figure 5–3). When athletes damage these ligaments, they often blame it on improper training, poor technique, fatigue, or bad luck. Nonathletes use the "accidents do happen" excuse.

Another of the usual suspects is supination and pronation, which I discussed in chapter 4. The reasoning goes this way: When a basketball player explosively pushes off with the outer edges of his or her feet—supinates—the pressure exceeds the ankle's tolerance. Likewise with pronation: As the leaping basketball player lands, the inside edge of the foot moves upward, perhaps because the player stepped on a competitor's foot, putting the ankle into a zone where damage will occur.

But as you recall from chapter 4, it isn't pronation and supination that causes the injury. The foot and ankle are designed to work on rough surfaces, but when the ankle is deprived of assistance from the arches of the foot below and the knee and hip above, it is left to take direct hit after direct hit. The "weak ankle" that one feels is the symptom of a joint that is pushing its limits as it twists and turns and wobbles with acute instability. It is also symptomatic of wider dysfunctions that involve failing arches and misaligned knee and hip load-bearing joints. Under the circumstances, the ankle's flexibility, one of its greatest assets, becomes a major liability.

In most sprains, the muscles and joints are pushed beyond their normal range of motion to produce trauma (usually swelling and tenderness), but the trauma stops short of out-and-out dislocation or ligament damage. When a ligament is involved, it tears parallel with its longitudinal fiber; while this is painful, the wider damage to the overall ankle itself is what's causing the bulk of the discomfort.

When the ankle is in pain, the temptation is to let the foot evert (turn out), but this will only put further nondesign stress on the injured ligaments and promote swelling. The heel-ball-toe gait allows the arches to engage, promotes knee interaction, and dampens the supinating and pronating tendencies that torque the joint from side

THE EGOSCUE METHOD TREATMENT FOR (NONFRACTURE) ANKLE PAIN

- After making sure that you are dealing with a sprain and not a fracture, plunge the ankle in ice water, and keep it submerged as long as you can stand it. When the cold becomes unbearable, come up for relief for a minute or two, then put it back in the water. Ten to twelve minutes of this in-and-out routine will combat swelling.
- Do the Supine Groin Stretch (page 72) for 35 to 45 minutes. It will realign the load-bearing joints on each side of the body and help reposition the ankle properly.
- Put on a sock and shoe, stand up, and gradually add weight to the ankle. When it is fully loaded, start walking again, carefully and slowly. *Make sure* your feet are pointed straight ahead and that as you walk, the foot's heel-ball-toe gait-pattern is occurring.
- Repeat the Supine Groin Stretch daily until the ankle is back to normal.

to side. Wrapping an Ace bandage around the ankle for a little extra support is okay, but you should avoid stiffer braces because they interfere with the heel-ball-toe gait and encourage the muscles of the inner thigh to take over, which undermines knee and hip functions.

Pay attention to your body. You will feel discomfort. If the pain is severe or escalates as you walk, don't push it too hard. Take frequent breathers. Sit down, elevate the ankle, and give it a rest. Still, it is important to get a load back on the joint as soon as possible. All muscles and joints lose function in direct proportion to lack of use.

Fractured Ankles

A fracture will require either surgery or manipulation by an orthopedic specialist to reunite the bones properly; there's no way around it. The healing process can be helped along, however, by the Supine Groin Stretch on page 72. All the hip and knee E-cises in subsequent chapters will help to realign those joints in preparation for the time when your doctor says it is okay to load and walk again on the injured ankle.

Surgery on a joint should be only a last resort. Screws and plates are strong, but the body, left to its own natural devices, is not only stronger but smarter. It was once common for medical practitioners to be able to maneuver the broken bones back into place without surgery, but unfortunately this is becoming a lost art. It's worth finding a physician who has the skill and experience to employ this less invasive technique, whenever it is appropriate.

The same basic treatment goes for dislocations and ruptured ligaments. In those cases, while there has been no bone fracture, the components of the ankle joint were violently disturbed and need to be allowed to resume their proper relationships and functions. In a remarkably short time, they will.

In fractures, sprains, and other musculoskeletal conditions, the swelling is usually less a reflection of actual localized damage than a measure of the stress and trauma that the surrounding tissue underwent when the accident took place. As such, the injury and the swelling are two different conditions. The best way to handle swelling is to work on restoring the hip-knee-ankle alignment. This will enhance the natural blood flow, help clear away injury-related waste products, and promote oxygenation of the area. The Supine Groin Stretch E-cise is effective in this respect because the injured structure is being aligned and engaged with the other joints without being loaded.

Swelling in the lower extremities can also have a serious internal source, like a heart problem or diabetes, so this advice applies only to swelling associated with musculoskeletal trauma.

Inflammation of the Achilles Tendon

The Achilles tendon got a bad rap thanks to Achilles' ambitious mother, who, according to legend, dipped her infant son in the magical waters of the river Styx to make him immortal. But the greatest of all the ancient Greek warriors had one small vulnerability: the heel of the foot by which his mother held him for his mythical baptism. It remained dry and unprotected. In the last days of the Trojan War, a spear hit that one spot, with the help of the god Apollo, and killed Achilles at the gates of Troy.

Homer, the author of this tale, knew human anatomy. Relatively narrow in diameter and unprotected by bone or muscle mass, the Achilles tendon is vulnerable not only to Trojan spear points but to the baseball spikes of a runner making a slide into second base.

In warfare the lower leg and foot cannot be as heavily armored as the upper torso, if the soldier is to have any mobility. But if not properly protected, the Achilles tendon of a combatant on horseback is easily slashed by an opponent on the ground. All of that is truly ancient history.

Although the Achilles tendon is not inherently vulnerable to injury, it is hurt more often than any other tendon. Why? For the same reason that the ankle joint itself takes such a beating: dysfunction. The Achilles tendon attaches the gastrocnemius muscle of the calf to the heel of the foot. Together, their job is to operate what amounts to the body's most powerful lever (figure 5–4). When we walk and run, our entire weight is heaved off the ground and moved forward by the gastrocnemius (and the soleus muscle) with the help of the Achilles tendon, which transmits the muscles' enormous power to the foot. Like its Greek namesake, the Achilles tendon is no wimp: Not surprisingly, considering the work it has to do, it is the most powerful tendon in the body.

Muscles work in opposition to other muscles: One flexes, another extends. The same rule of opposition is true of tendons. The Achilles tendon's opposing tendons anchor the two heads of the gastrocnemius muscle to the medial and lateral malleolus of the femur (the twin knobs at the end of the bone that form part of the knee joint). But one of these tendons originates at a spot that is slightly lower than the other, which means that any knee misalignment will disrupt the dynamic tension and interaction of the tendons. The Achilles tendon, instead of delivering a taut, smooth contraction, starts twanging or crimping. To visualize this, imagine holding the opposite ends of a rolled-up dish towel in your right and left hands. Keeping the towel straight and tight and simultaneously moving your hands to the left and right resembles the Achilles tendon's healthy contraction-relaxation mechanism. Now, keep the right hand in place while moving the left back and forth: The towel folds and droops. This is what happens to the Achilles tendon when the knee is misaligned.

The Achilles tendon was not designed to "twang," or to move an unstable pronating and supinating foot with compromised arches, least of all without much help from other opposing muscles of the lower leg, knee, or hip. The tendon's contractile force is such that it is capable of suddenly moving a load that is many times the body's weight; and yet that same strength, when turned against itself, is extremely damaging. For one thing, it can cause inflammation; worse, constant friction from an imbalance between the Achilles tendon and its opposing tendon may produce a painful large callus on

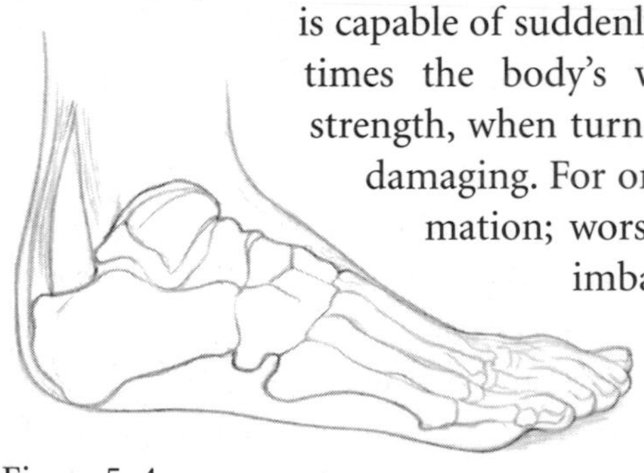

Figure 5–4
The attachment of the Achilles tendon to the heel.

SIX ACHILLES TENDON DANGER SIGNS

1. Do your shoes wear unevenly?
2. Are your feet everted when you stand or walk?
3. If you gently pinch along the length of your Achilles tendon, is it tender?
4. Sit down with your leg straight out and propped on the edge of a desk. When you flex your foot toward you, do you feel the action in your ankle? (You should feel it in the calf.)
5. In the same position, when the foot flexes, does the inside edge lead the way and the outside follow at an angle?
6. Do your calf muscles feel unusually tight most of the time?

---

the back of the ankle. Many physicians treat such a callus by scraping and paring it down. This makes it easier to walk without pain, but it does nothing to address the cause of the problem, so it will probably recur. Moreover, the tendon is weakened by the procedure. E-cise therapy is far more effective. Outright rupture of the tendon, however, requires surgery.

All sorts of special techniques have been devised to protect the Achilles tendon, from special warm-up and stretching routines to avoiding cinder tracks and other playing surfaces deemed potentially hazardous. The best precaution of all, however, is prevention, by eliminating musculoskeletal dysfunctions that may be endangering your Achilles tendon.

Four E-cises for Achilles Tendon Pain (or its Prevention)

Total time: Thirty minutes.
Times a day: Once in the morning.
Duration: Do exercises daily until pain abates for

twenty-four hours. Once the pain is gone, continue with
the menu for one week before switching to the overall
conditioning program in chapter 13.

- FOOT CIRCLES

Follow the routine for Foot Circles in chapter 4 (figure 4–5, page
53). Be sure to circle both feet, even though the Achilles tendon
pain is on only one side. Foot Circles remind the ankle of its
design range of motion. Do not do the Point Flexes.

- STATIC BACK
  (Figure 5–5)

Lie on your back, with both legs bent at right angles on a chair or
block. Rest your hands on your stomach or the floor, below
shoulder level, with palms up. Let the back settle into the floor.

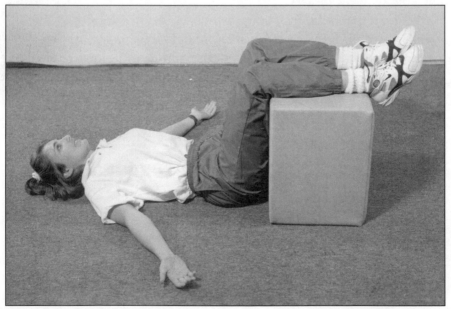

Figure 5–5

Breathe from your diaphragm (that is, do stomach breathing). The abdominal muscles should rise as you inhale and fall as you exhale. Hold this position for five to ten minutes. This E-cise will settle the hips to the floor and release the compensating muscles that are interfering with the gait-pattern of the foot and ankle.

- STATIC WALL
  (Figure 5–6)

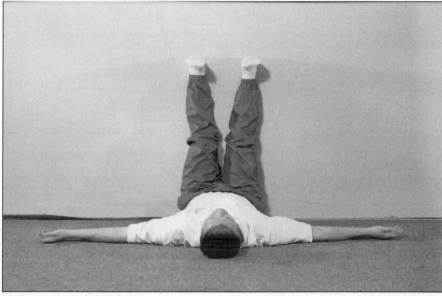

Figure 5–6

Lie on your back. Place your legs straight up against the wall hip-width apart. Tighten your thighs, and flex your feet and toes back toward the floor. Get your buttocks and hamstrings (the posterior of the thigh) as close to the wall as you can. The smaller the gap, the better. Concentrate on relaxing your upper body. Hold for three to five minutes. Static Wall engages the anterior muscles of the thighs and lower legs.

● **Supine Groin Stretch**
(Figure 5–7)

This E-cise tames the powerful muscles that run along the inside
of your thighs. Lie on your back with one leg resting on a block or
chair, the knee bent at a ninety-degree angle, while the other leg is
extended straight out and resting on the floor. Make sure that
both legs are aligned with the hips and shoulders. The foot of the
extended leg should be propped upright to prevent it from rolling
to one side. Relax in this position for at least ten minutes, then
switch sides.

An alternative way to time this E-cise is to use the thigh test.
Contract the thigh of the extended leg, and determine where you
feel the strongest part of the contraction. Initially it will be near
the knee. As the stretch continues, do the test contractions every

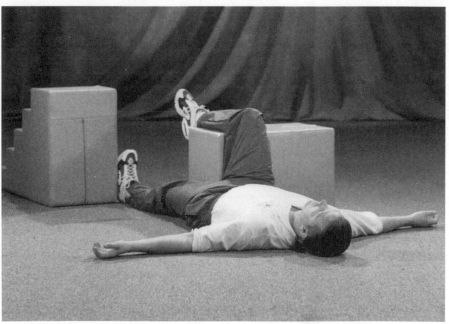

Figure 5–7

three to five minutes; the strongest part will move up the thigh. Don't hold the thigh in contraction; simply contract it and release it for the test. When you feel the contraction at the top of the thigh, it's time to switch sides.

A Quick Calf Roundup

The calves consist of five muscles, two in what's known as the superficial flexor layer and three more underneath them in the deep flexor layer. They are as uncomplicated as they are powerful.

Without the mighty muscles of the calf, it would be next to impossible to achieve or sustain upright posture. Not only are they essential for locomotion, but when we are on our feet they are constantly fighting gravity to prevent the body from toppling forward. I said standing would be "next to impossible" without powerful calves because dysfunctions and the resulting musculoskeletal compensation reassign the calves' responsibility to the knees, inner thighs, and low back. These mechanisms end up battling gravity, which is a losing fight. The calves, meanwhile, atrophy (but retain just enough power to damage the Achilles tendon).

It's one reason that calf implants are among the most common surgical silicone-implant procedures. Weight lifters, for instance, after spending hours in the gym buffing their upper torsos, are sometimes driven nuts by their flaccid and puny calf muscles. They *bomb* their calves with a variety of exercises and machines, all to no avail. This happens—or doesn't happen—because the muscles are not receiving regular stimulus after the athlete leaves the weight room. His routine calf functions are usurped by the muscles of the thighs, hips, and low back, which are being stimulated by a modern lifestyle that uses them for such purposes as sitting down and the small amount of walking that's required to get the individual from chair to chair. With feet everted and knees rotated, the calves switch off the moment the special exercise regimen ends and start losing whatever strength they've gained. The weight lifters turn to the implants as a last resort—forgetting, of course, that the *first resort* works every time: restoring function. Those flabby calf muscles are out of the loop thanks to dysfunction. They can't respond because the stimulus isn't reaching them. Development of the calf muscles depends on the proper alignment of all four pairs of the load-bearing joints.

Shin Splints

You may have thought that shin splints have nothing to do with calves. But if you bring proper motion to the calves, your shin splints will disappear.

Shin splints are actually the most painful condition involving the calves. With each running step, they feel as if the muscle tissue on the front of the leg above the ankle is tearing. And, basically, that is what's happening. As the feet and ankles attempt to perform their lever-and-hinge function in the presence of excessive pronation, supination, and lateral torque (take your pick), the sheathing of the anterior muscles of the lower leg suffer minute tears. Just imagine the lower leg twisting, gyrating, and vibrating as it runs, instead of smoothly extending and flexing; the muscle sheathing is being subjected to ferocious abuse. Once again, getting new shoes, using orthotics, running on a different surface, and taking up a low-impact sport are the wrong answers to the right question.

> **Unevenly worn shoes do not cause shin splints. Shin splints cause unevenly worn shoes.**

The question, of course, is how do I stop the pain? And the right answer involves using these E-cises to correct improper foot strike, which was discussed in chapter 4. The following E-cises are designed to restore coordinated movement among the hips, knees, and ankles, in order to allow the muscle sheathing to heal.

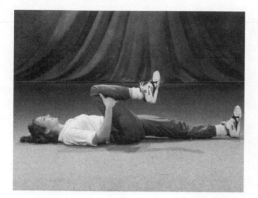

- FOOT CIRCLES AND POINT FLEXES

Follow the instructions for this E-cise in chapter 4 (figure 4–5, page 53).

- SUPINE CALF/HAMSTRING STRETCH WITH A STRAP

Follow the instructions for this E-cise in chapter 4 (figures 4–6a and 4–6b, page 54).

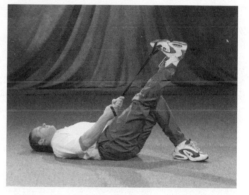

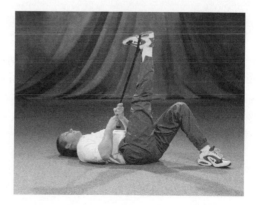

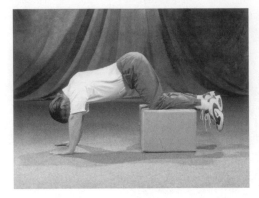

• STATIC EXTENSION

Follow the instructions for this E-cise in chapter 4 (figure 4–7, page 56).

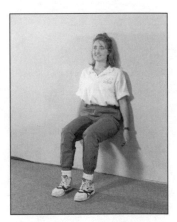

• AIR BENCH

Follow the instructions for this E-cise in chapter 4 (figure 4–8, page 57).

Cramps

If you have frequent cramps in your calves, it's most likely a reaction to having the muscles do work they are unaccustomed to doing. Dehydration and poor nutrition are also likely factors. It will help to refrain from drinking beverages that contain stimulants. Stick to water, and consume a lot of it. No E-cise is necessary for cramps; try gently massaging and kneading the cramped area and flexing the foot toward the knee. Like all chronic pain, cramps in the lower legs are telling you something important. Stop, look, and listen.

KNEES: GOOD NEWS ABOUT BAD KNEES

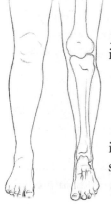

Figure 6 1

The knee is a complex joint that does a simple job: synchronizing the hip and ankle. I could easily reverse the statement and say that the knee is a simple joint doing a complex job. Both are true.

The knee is also an elegant solution to a fiendishly difficult problem. The hip and ankle move at vastly different rates of speed; their gears, if you will, vary in size. Their muscular power sources range from the equivalent of jet propulsion to rubber bands. Hooking them up together is at once madness and pure genius. When it happened, sometime prior to 3.2 million years ago, our ancestors found the strength, stamina, agility, and speed to compete with the four-legged creatures of greater size and ferocity that, until then, had ruled the earth.

Knee Injuries Grow More Common Among the Young

I get exasperated when I hear how "fragile" knees are. If that's the case, why aren't human beings extinct as a species? If our knees couldn't handle crawling, walking, running, jumping, and falling down—routine physical demands—we'd have gone out of business several thousand years ago. The design is the same today as it was then.

"But," the argument goes, "humankind is living longer. Knees are programmed to give out after the child-bearing and child-rearing ages." If that were true, logically it would also be true for all the other major components of the musculoskeletal system, and we'd have only extremely rare instances of breakdown prior to age forty or forty-five. But in my clinic we are starting to see more teenagers and young adults with knee problems than older or late middle-aged clients. And the numbers and ratio appear to be growing. Granted, the clinic may not attract a representative sample of the general population. But if anything, it would be skewed toward older individuals. Yet those in their fifties to their eighties tend to have less severe biomechanical dysfunctions and more overall joint stability than younger people. Frankly, the young people we see are a mess.

It's an ominous development. As musculoskeletal breakdown occurs at earlier and earlier ages, we may be moving toward a major physiological crisis. We can't count on technology to provide total mobility, or even adequate partial mobility, to the functionally immobile. Furthermore, the body's metabolic system will not properly function without adequate motion.

When I see young men and women, even girls and boys, with bad knees, I think of the canaries that eighteenth- and nineteenth-century coal miners took into the mines to detect gas seepage. Small traces would kill them in midsong. The resulting silence was like a clanging alarm bell, warning the miners to clear out. Similarly, these dysfunctions are warning us of danger. Lose the ability in youth to synchronize the hip and the knee, and we are on the way to forfeiting locomotion itself.

Accidents Don't Just Happen

Healthy knees need only one thing: alignment with the other load-bearing joints. Knees rarely have problems if they are aligned and allowed to work in association with the ankles and hips. But we've persuaded ourselves that knees are accidents waiting to happen, time bombs ready to explode at any moment. Accidents and explosions do happen, although I regard them in this context as *symptomatic events*. Damaging a patella when suddenly stopping to change direction on a soccer field or tearing the anterior cruciate ligament (ACL) during a tumble while skiing are misconstrued as misfortunes, mishaps, and misadventures. They may be all of those things and more, but they cause damage to the knee only in a secondary sense, much as a hammer *causes* a careless carpenter's broken thumb. If the knee had been aligned, the soccer player would have stopped

---

PATELLA AND ACL

The patella is the kneecap, a disk of bone that seems to float freely atop the joint. Actually, it is embedded in the tendons of the extensor muscles of the leg. This arrangement gives the knee a lot of flexibility. The anterior cruciate ligament (ACL) is a tough band of tissue that crisscrosses the knee joint from the rear to give it stability.

---

on a dime, turned, kicked, and scored the goal, while the skier would have dusted off the snow and continued hot-dogging down the hill.

It is essential to escape from this "accidents do happen" fixation; the E-cises in this chapter will help you do that, but first we've all got to reexamine our assumptions about the causes of pain. If we are convinced that pain is the result of an isolated accident and a vulnerable joint, we will mistakenly believe that just fixing the damage is enough. Since knees are damaged more than any other joint, a whole industry has developed to service them and eliminate pain. Knee surgery is the Midas muffler of orthopedics. Repair the joint—or replace it—and move on.

Physicians, being human, are not immune to buying into the assumptions that the rest of us make. We go to doctors to relieve pain, they oblige us, then they see the next patient. Gradually, they lose track of the cause-and-effect relationship because the effect—chronic musculoskeletal pain—returns in different forms accompanied by different symptomatic events, or "causes." Instead of skiing, the victim was playing squash, and he or she smashed up a shoulder. The logical circle has been broken. The doctor dutifully fixes the shoulder and never makes the connection between the two episodes because *accidents happen*. Besides, *knees are fragile.*

> ## WHICH COMES FIRST, THE ACCIDENT OR THE DYSFUNCTION?
>
> Symptomatic events are variable: slipping in the shower, tripping over a crack in the sidewalk, falling on the tennis court, and so on. What is constant is the knee dysfunction that existed *prior* to the event and the inevitable damage it causes sooner or later.

Almost every client who comes to my clinic is a refugee from this crazed geometric progression that starts with a minor dysfunctional condition and carries on from symptomatic event to symptomatic event right to the brink of catastrophe. Terry Cantor was a classic case. In his mid-forties he was unable to fully straighten out his right knee, a condition that persisted for twelve more years until he came to the clinic in 1997.

Terry's Story

When I first saw Terry, he had had surgery on both his rotator cuffs, an operation on the right knee to remove damaged cartilage, and his doctors wanted to replace the left knee.

Terry's problems had started after he began to feel an unusual tightness in his left hip. Back then, he was an equipment salesman, traveling by car from customer to customer. He spent hours on the road, his right leg resting against the fire wall of his car, operating the accelerator. His left leg was more active as it worked the clutch. When he stopped to get out, he used his left leg and the rest of that side to pull himself out of the driver's seat.

It didn't take long for the left side to overpower the right. The stronger left hip contributed to pulling the weaker right hip down and toward the posterior.

The pelvis is truly the body's foundation. Its great utility comes in part from the ability to flex and reposition itself in response to the powerful muscular forces of the back and thighs.

Even so, the pelvis is intended to always return to its bilateral, vertically aligned starting point. But Terry's weak right-side muscles couldn't hold their side of the pelvis in proper position. As he walked from the parking lot to the customers' office to make a sales call, his right knee was being forced to operate out of phase with the hip. The pelvic alignment was not there; nor was the required dynamic interaction. The kinetic chain linking the shoulder, hip, knee, and ankle had been broken.

All joints are built to rotate. This means that in addition to hinging like a door, joints have a certain amount of lateral movement as well. In this respect, they resemble a gimbal, a device that keeps a ship's compass level, as the vessel pitches and rolls with the waves, by allowing it to swing freely in any direction. Of course, unlike a gimbal, the joints' range of motion is restricted; otherwise they wouldn't be able to perform the task of vertical load-bearing (or keep from collapsing into a heap of bones and muscles whenever we bend over to tie our shoes).

Every joint thus has a certain amount of internal and external *play* built into it to accommodate rotational demand. We use joint rotation to twist and turn suddenly, bob and weave, and stretch and straddle. However, compared with flexion and extension—lifting the leg off the ground and then stepping down with the foot—the amount of rotational leeway in the knee is limited.

Unfortunately, Terry was using all of it, and more, with every step he took. His knee was trying to move him forward on a straight line, but since it was not aligned with the hip, it lacked the biome-

---

THE BODY BILATERAL

Except for the spine and skull, the human musculoskeletal system has two of everything. Both halves of the body, to the left and right of the spine, are functionally identical. Both sides are designed to operate in the same manner. When they don't, the balance and health of the entire system are affected.

chanical capacity to do that job without using extra rotation, accompanied by muscular improvisation and compensation.

When Terry sensed that something was wrong, he decided to "get in shape" by running and working out on the exercise machines at the gym. In fact, he was active physically whenever he took time away from the job. But a few hours of physical activity on the weekends cannot counteract days of what I call *patterned motion*—get in the car, drive, climb out, walk, get back in the car, drive, and so on. Once Terry's body went unilateral, a muscular imbalance set in, with knee, hip, and ankle rotation and muscular compensation from the adductors and abductors (muscles that move body parts laterally toward and away from the medial line).

Thus, since he did not first realign his knees and other load-bearing joints with patterned-motion-breaking E-cises, his exercising ended up reinforcing his dysfunctions. The workout that was supposed to make him feel better was really furthering long-term damage to his knee and other mechanisms. And the key word is *long-term*. This is what causes chronic pain.

Time + Trauma = Pain

The impressive thing about the body's design is that it is built to tolerate violations of its standard operating procedure. We can work ourselves into amazing postures, positions, and contortions, as the more advanced yoga masters prove time and again. They get away with it because they leave the kinetic chain that links the ankles, knees, hips, and shoulders intact. Break that chain of alignment and interaction, and leave it broken for months and years, and the accumulated damage becomes too much to bear. A new chain takes its place: a chain reaction of dysfunction and pain.

To stabilize his right knee, Terry began unconsciously shifting his weight to his left side. It was a way of ensuring balance. His left hip, knee, leg, and foot (each in isolation) ended up doing extra work and pounding into the ground harder. Since his left hip was out of position posteriorly, he brought his upper torso forward by

bending slightly at the waist, then led with the left shoulder to compensate for the disengaged hip. This, in effect, took the props out
from under his shoulders; his skeletal structure started to sag forward and down. As his shoulder muscles and the muscles of his upper back and neck struggled with his new head position and the
drooping shoulder yoke, they were forced to tighten up.

Imagine two horizontal lines drawn through the hips and
shoulders. Seen from the front, Terry's hips were rotating counterclockwise, while the upper torso was rotating
clockwise. In addition, since his weight had
shifted to the left, that shoulder was elevated
to help brace the load-bearing side of the
body, while the right dropped back to act as a
counterweight against the head. The center
of gravity, meanwhile, shifted from directly over the ankles toward the balls
of the feet (figure 6–2).

You are looking at a problem that
is not unique to Terry. Millions of
people have lost their horizontal integrity and vertical load-bearing ability. Sensing that he is about to fall
over, Terry's flexor-extensor muscles
(which are also the main posture muscles) have locked up to various degrees.
Meanwhile, other muscles involved in
rotation, abduction, and adduction are
working furiously to keep him mobile
and upright. These muscles are not primarily posture muscles; they have other
specialties, such as accomplishing lateral
movement and allowing a wide range of
adjustments within a joint. Now, however, they are also being forced to
keep the body upright. Over time,
the accumulated stress and damage
caused by this nondesign motion

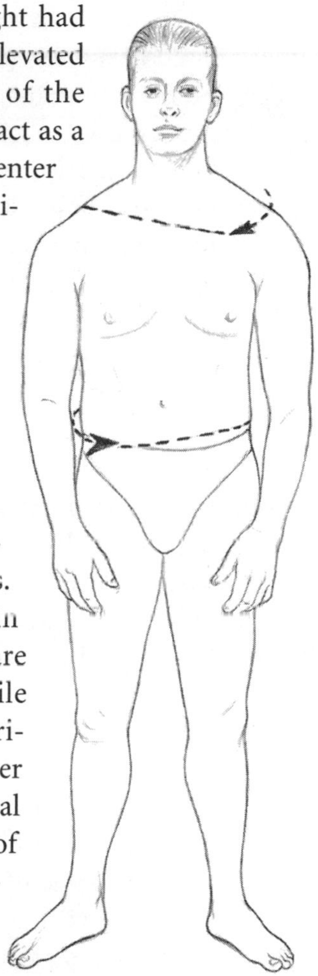

Figure 6–2

Misaligned shoulders and hips.

causes the surrogate or substitute posture flexor-extensors to go into constant (or sporadic) contraction.

Is it any wonder that the cartilage in the knees wears away? Is it any wonder that the rotator cuffs of the shoulder are tight or that they tear when the inevitable symptomatic event comes along?

Terry's doctors explained to him that he had damaged his right knee cartilage in a fall and that arthritis was compounding the problem. They went in and removed the damaged cartilage, but afterward Terry was unable to straighten his right knee fully. This nasty surprise should have been predictable since, by removing damaged cartilage, the doctors reduced the glide surface that the excessively rotating joint had used to fully straighten the knee. But the pain was gone—and that was priority number one.

Years later, and only after the rotator cuff repairs and the announcement that he needed a left knee replacement, did Terry realize that priority number one was not pain abatement. The doctors said the knee replacement would make him pain free, but he would have to curtail all of his favorite sports and physical activities. He decided he couldn't live that way, and he was right: He was killing himself with the very means he had chosen to kill the pain.

Terry decided not to have surgery after the knee, the one that he had been unable to fully straighten for twelve years, returned to full function after a three-hour session in the Egoscue Method Clinic. A series of E-cises—most of them from the menu in this chapter—released his tight left pelvic girdle muscles and allowed his hips to return to a neutral position instead of putting rotation into the knee. When Terry finished the last item on his therapy menu, he got up off the floor and almost fell over. The sensation of having a straight knee was so strange and unexpected, he had almost forgotten how to stand on two feet with a functional knee.

During the course of his treatment, Terry learned how to look at his knees and the rest of his body. He realized that he had been bearing a disproportionate amount of weight on the left side, which allowed him to make the cause-and-effect linkage. The effect was knee pain.

KNEES AND GENDER

The newspapers and magazines have discovered knees—particularly women's knees. A lot is being written about how female athletes are more likely than males to damage the anterior cruciate ligament in their knees. This is ascribed to musculoskeletal differences between men and women. But the knee and the ACL are exactly the same for both sexes. Women have more flexion-extension capability in the pelvis to allow for childbirth, but this attribute isn't responsible for ACL ruptures.

Sexual inequality is to blame. Women are entering sports without benefit of the kind of physical conditioning programs that are readily available to men. Putting a woman on a basketball court and asking her to play hard is fine, but she also needs to be given the opportunity and the time off the court to develop the appropriate musculature and functions from head to foot—not just strength training, aerobics, or sport-specific drills. Those functions are equally accessible to men and women who understand that athletic success comes from working with, not against, the design of the body.

The Ins and Outs of Knee Pain

Long ago, I gave up counting the number of individual knee maladies. Patellofemoral disease, meniscitis, prepatellar bursitis, knee osteoarthritis, chondromalacia patellae, locked knee—whatever the knee malady, it is directly related to what is happening in the other load-bearing joints.

Yes, there may be cartilage damage.

Yes, there may be a damaged ligament.

Yes, there may be a Baker's cyst behind the knee or some other painful problem.

And yes, each condition can be treated with surgical procedures and drugs. But in each case the cause of the real knee problem will remain untreated.

Stand in front of a full-length mirror wearing a pair of shorts (shoes off), and look at your knees. Don't try to straighten your feet; stand naturally. Wiggle a little to get loose. Functional knees are lined up directly under the hips and above the ankles. Imagine a straight line. Better yet, try what we do in the clinic: Take a marking pen, and draw a big blue dot on the middle of each kneecap and another set on the front of the ankles. If you have a dysfunction, the knees will be either on the inside or on the outside of an invisible line that runs vertically between the dots. If you back up and then walk toward the mirror, you will probably see the dots gyrate wildly—now inside, then outside the line—and in a different sequence for the right and left sides and for all four joints. What's happening? The better question is, what's *not* happening? Proper synchronization is not happening.

The starting point of a completely pain-free knee is a completely bilateral body. To turn pain off, we must restore the affected body part to a neutral position. Proper bilateral function will create balance where dysfunction created a muscular tug-of-war. Without bilateral function, muscles pull on bones and other muscles, tendons, connective tissues, and nerves. At minimum, this is stressful, but it also causes an actual rearrangement of the musculoskeletal system that ultimately results in accumulating physical disability, pain, and far-reaching physiological disruption.

Aside from pain, the two most recognizable symptoms of knee problems appear in the feet and the kneecaps. Everted feet are evidence that the kinetic chain linking the ankles, knees, hips, and shoulders has been broken. The knees are on their own. In many cases, only one foot will be turned out, or both will turn, but at different angles. It depends on what the individual is trying to do with the dysfunctional body.

After you've tried this exercise, stop in front of the mirror and examine your kneecaps closely. A functional kneecap points straight ahead. Yours may be pointing in the direction of your everted feet,

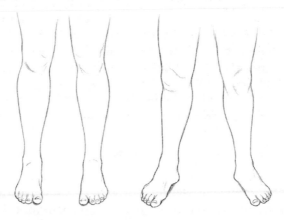

Figure 6–3
Functional and dysfunctional knees.

or aiming off at a totally different angle. Again, the two kneecaps may not match up at all: One could be higher than the other, twisted medially or laterally, or have a markedly different shape (figure 6–3). In a bilateral body, the right side resembles the left side. Mismatches tell us that unilateral processes are under way, and your knees are on their own. Rather than tracking at ninety degrees while flexing and extending, rotating slightly and returning to neutral, the bones are being jerked around by improvising muscles. There's tightness, stiffness, sometimes a sense of weakness and, finally, pain. This ultimate symptom can vary from a mild and intermittent pain, to throbbing and acute pain that persuades you not to bend the knee at all.

Whatever the symptom, please observe this rule:

Avoid preventive knee bracing.

Bracing any body part restricts its movement, and that does more damage in the long run by making the muscles and joints less capable of moving properly. A knee brace changes the interaction between the joint and the conjoined bones—the tibia, fibula, and fe-

A word about *quads,* or two words actually: Forget them. Entirely too much fuss has been made about strengthening the quads to protect the knee. They will take care of themselves if the hip is stabilized. If it is not, working on the quads is a total waste of time. The weak pelvic girdle muscles that left the pelvis in flexion have to contend with the beefed-up quads that are performing—guess what?—an extensor muscle role.

mur. The thighbone, the femur, the body's most formidable long bone, reacts to the brace by changing its pattern of motion in the hip joint socket. Believe me, you don't want that to happen—serious hip and back problems can result. With a brace, you're piling dysfunction on top of dysfunction. It only seems to make your knee feel more stable. What you are actually feeling is immobility, and an immobile joint is a dying joint.

Knee Pain: Internal Rotation

When we work with knee pain at the clinic, we initially look for only two primary conditions that may be causing it. The first condition is internal rotation of the knee (toward the inside of the leg). This condition is usually the easiest to identify (figure 6–4). In its most

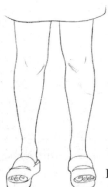

pronounced form, the individual looks knock-kneed. What's going on is that the muscles of the pelvic girdle are weak, which makes the pelvis stay in flexion, losing its ability to extend. As a result, the femur is rotated inward with each step, as adductor muscles pull the leg back toward the trunk of the body. As a result of the lost extension of the pelvis, the femur doesn't have sufficient counterrotation.

Figure 6–4
Knees with internal rotation.

> Total time: This menu can take a while because of the Supine Groin Stretch on Towels. For severe pain, you may want to do this stretch for forty-five minutes to an hour. For slight pain, fifteen to twenty minutes will do.
>
> Times a day: Once in the morning.
>
> Duration: Do exercises daily until pain abates for twenty-four hours. Once the pain is gone, continue with the menu for one week before switching to the overall conditioning program in chapter 13.

Here are the E-cises that I recommend for internal rotation:

- STANDING GLUTEAL CONTRACTIONS
  (Figure 6–5 a and b)

Stand up straight, hands at your sides. Squeeze your buttocks together; be sure to use the buttock muscles, not the thighs or abdominals. Do one set with your feet straight, hip-width apart,

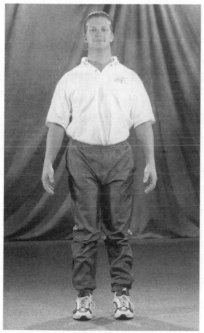

Figure 6–5a

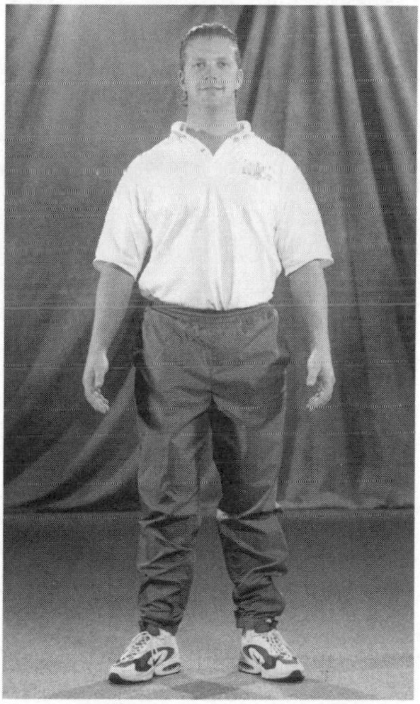

Figure 6–5b

and one set with your feet everted (out), hip-width apart; do three
sets of twenty repetitions.

We sit on our gluteals so much, they atrophy. This E-cise is a
quick and easy way to get them back in action.

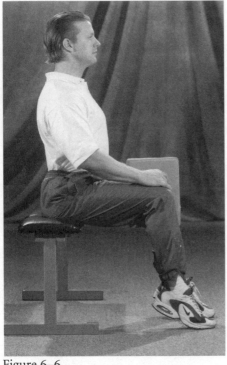

Figure 6–6

• SITTING HEEL RAISES
(Figure 6–6)

Sit on the edge of a chair or
bench, and arch your low back by
rolling your hips forward. Place a
pillow or foam block between
your knees, and simultaneously lift your heels off the floor. The
toes remain in contact with the floor throughout and pointed
straight ahead. Raise your heels. Don't push off the toes; instead,
use the hip flexor muscles. Imagine that your toes are resting on
eggshells; do three sets of fifteen repetitions.

It's amazing what muscular improvisation goes on simply to
flex and extend the foot when there is dysfunction. This E-cise
short-circuits all of it.

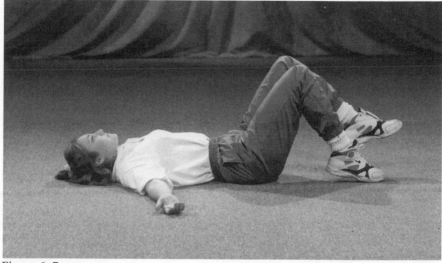

Figure 6–7

- ISOLATED HIP FLEXOR LIFTS ON A TOWEL
  (Figure 6–7)

Lie on your back with your knees bent, feet flat on the floor. Use
two towels, each rolled to about a three-and-a-half-inch diameter.
Put one behind your neck, the other under the arch of your low
back just above the hips. The idea is to offer support, not to
elevate the hips or head. Lift one foot three to four inches off the
floor. Keep the knee in line with the shoulders and the foot in line
with the knee. Do three sets of ten repetitions. Repeat on the
other side.

In this routine, the knee and the foot ascend as the hip flexors
(in the front of the hip), not the abdominals or thighs, do the
work.

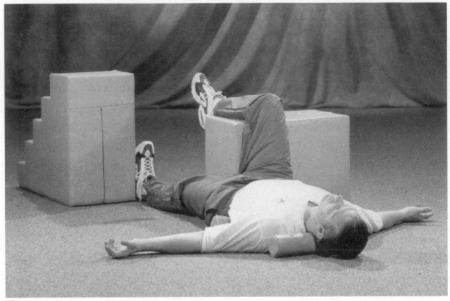

Figure 6–8

- SUPINE GROIN STRETCH ON TOWELS
  (Figure 6–8)

Lie on your back with one leg resting on a block, knee bent at a
ninety-degree angle, while the other leg is extended straight out
and resting on the floor. Put rolled towels (about three and a half
inches in diameter) under your neck and low back. Prop upright
the foot of the extended leg to prevent it from rolling out to one
side. Hold until the extended leg is completely relaxed, then
reverse the legs and repeat. Use the thigh test described for the
Supine Groin Stretch (figure 5–7, page 72), for the best timing
results. At first, it could take as long as forty-five minutes a side to
release the hold the groin muscles have on the leg.

Knee Pain: External Rotation

The second primary knee condition that we look for as a cause of knee pain is external rotation (the knee rotates outward). This condition can be harder to spot on your own (figure 6–9). If you have any doubt as to whether it is internal or external, assume that it is external rotation. The pain is caused because the pelvic girdle muscles are too tight. Generally, the pelvis is being held in extension, and the femur is being subjected to constant rotational torque toward the outside of the leg.

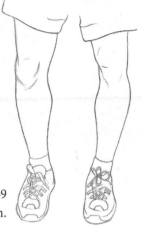

Figure 6–9
A knee with external rotation.

The E-cises are:

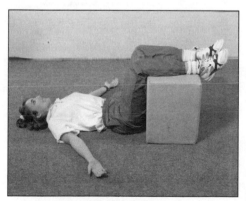

• STATIC BACK

This is the same E-cise as the Static Back in chapter 5 (figure 5–5, page 70). It has been a mainstay in the clinic for years. Gravity puts the left and right hips flat into the floor. The structures of the hips and trunk work best, and according to design, when they are on the same plane. This E-cise puts them there.

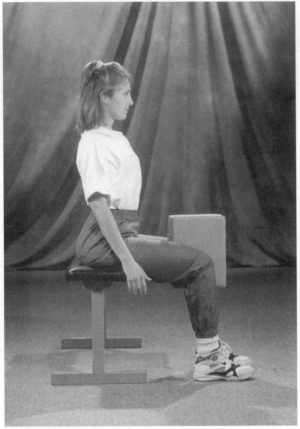

Figure 6–10

• SITTING KNEE
  PILLOW SQUEEZES
  (Figure 6–10)

Sit on the edge of a chair or bench, and arch your back by rolling your hips forward. Pull your shoulders back, and make sure your knees and feet are in alignment with your hips. Relax your stomach muscles; let them hang. Place a pillow between your knees, and using your inner thighs, squeeze the pillow and release it gently. You may need to fold the pillow to give it thickness. Your feet stay parallel to each other; and don't let your stomach or upper back participate. Do four sets of ten repetitions. The abductor and adductor muscles are doing their primary assignment, instead of trying to operate as gait muscles.

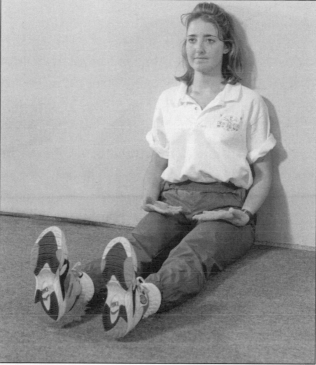

Figure 6–11

- SITTING FLOOR
  (Figure 6–11)

Sit against a wall with your legs straight out in front of you. Squeeze your shoulder blades together, and hold. Do not elevate your shoulders. Tighten the thighs and flex the feet so that the toes are pointing back toward you. Keep your arms at your sides or relaxed atop the thighs. Hold for four to six minutes. This E-cise establishes a shoulder, hip, knee, and ankle link.

- PROGRESSIVE SUPINE GROIN
  (Figure 6–12 a and b)

Lie on your back with one leg resting on a block or chair, knee bent at a ninety-degree angle, while the other leg is extended and elevated on a small stepladder, stack of books, or something similar, high enough that the back and hips are flat on the floor. The foot is resting on the heel. In the photo, the model's foot is resting about two feet in the air, but how high your foot goes will depend on your size. *Prop the foot of the extended leg on the outside to prevent it from rolling out.*

The idea is to progressively lower the extended foot about five to eight inches at a time until it rests on the floor. As you lower the leg, relax your back into the floor. Don't try to flatten your back—let it happen naturally. Hold this position at each step for a

Figure 6–12a

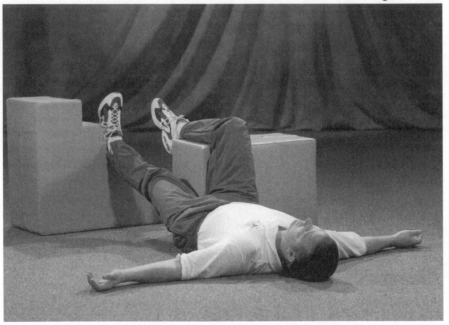

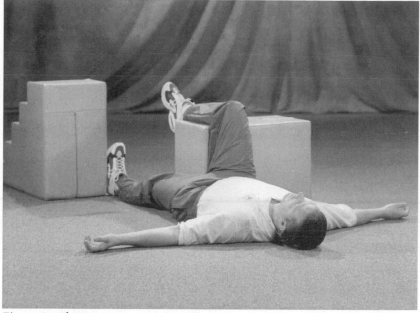

Figure 6–12b

minimum of three minutes. Repeat on the opposite side. The thigh test that we used for the Supine Groin Stretch (figure 5–7, page 72) is a good timing guide here, too.

This E-cise is designed to allow flexion and extension of the leg, rather than rotation through adduction and abduction (side-to-side movement).

Look at your knees—a lot! Constantly, if you are feeling pain. Signs of function or dysfunction are there to be seen. Our unique system of bipedal locomotion was designed to be self-diagnosing. Knees either look healthy and functional or they don't; there is an objective visual standard. Now that you understand how well designed and strong the knee is, you'll be able to spot the potential for accidents *before* they happen. Prevention is what being pain free is all about.

HIPS: UNITED WE STAND

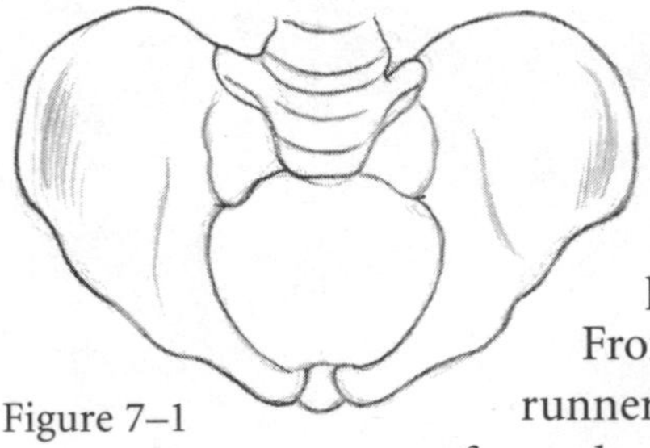

Figure 7–1

Located in the middle of the anatomical action, the hips are magnificent joints, key parts of the pelvic girdle. They unite two powerful creatures into one being. From the waist down, humans are runners and jumpers, high kickers, and fancy dancers. We spring, sprint, and stand still. From the waist up, we throw, climb hand-over-hand, bear heavy burdens, and grasp the tools and instruments of craft, art, and science.

As science writer Colin Tudge suggests in his book *The Time Before History,* this duality produced a centaurlike life-form, although without the encumbrance of the quadrupedal horse's half. Joined at the hips, humans became the first big predators who were capable of roaming the entire world on two feet and at the same time of killing at a distance by using two strong arms to throw weapons at their prey. All this was made possible by a no-frills, no-fuss pelvis that has a minimum of moving parts and a maximum of strength and flexibility. Unlike the instantly recognizable skull or rib cage, in skeletal form the pelvis looks scarcely human. Yet it is arguably the most characteristically human structure of the body. All vertebrates, for instance, have backbones, but none of them were lucky enough to get anything quite like our pelvis.

Solid as a . . . Hip

The pelvic girdle is, first and foremost, the linchpin of our upright posture. Without the pelvis as a *platform* and *fulcrum,* the spine would be horizontal. Like any platform that offers a stable and flat surface, the pelvis supports the spine from below. As a fulcrum, it also gives the spine leverage, a point from which it can be hoisted upright.

The pelvis unites the musculoskeletal components of the upper and lower halves of the body, but it also creates a jackknife effect. Once the body is fully extended and upright, the pelvis does not lock it into that position. Rather, like the blade of a jackknife, it can bend and straighten. The torso can also turn almost 180 degrees, thanks to the pelvis: It would be impossible to get into that position using only torso muscles or only hip and leg muscles (though a dysfunctional individual tries mightily).

This ability to turn makes the pelvis-fulcrum more than a glorified hinge, and the pelvis-platform more than a bowl-shaped anchor and point of origin for a bunch of muscles. Rather, it resembles a central steering or balancing mechanism. It is not too far-fetched to say that the pelvis is the body's other brain—that's how important it is. Judged by the amount of armored plating that nature has provided, the skull and the pelvis are definitely in the same league. Like the skull, the hip is built to endure incredible punishment while safeguarding essential functions.

Yet hip pain has become relatively common. Most of it is blamed on aging. Alerted by pain or stiffness, doctors take a look at the area where the head of the femur (the thighbone) inserts into the socket of the hip joint (figure 7–2). If they find inflammation and/or cartilage deterioration, they usually diagnose the condition as arthritis. The word *arthritis* spooks people, but it only means what it is objectively denoting in Latin—inflammation of a joint. In addition to the cartilage that coats the head of the femur, the hip joint also has an interior lining. Known as the synovium, this delicate membrane secretes a fluid that acts as a lubricant. This is the mechanism that, in arthritis, gets inflamed (swollen),

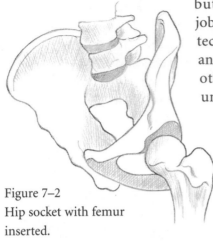

Figure 7–2

Hip socket with femur
inserted.

but actually it is only doing its job. The synovium is there to protect the joint, and when there is an unusual amount of friction or other irritation, it generates an unusual amount of fluid. There isn't much room in the joint; the extra lubricant gradually turns milky and viscous and restricts the ball-and-socket function.

Again, the synovium is guiltless. Swelling is a perfectly reasonable way to stop the joint from damaging itself. Its operation is much like that of an air bag, albeit one that deploys slowly, over the course of years rather than seconds. When musculoskeletal dysfunction is present, irritation of the synovium isn't a disease, and it isn't related to aging. Rather, the inflammation is caused by misalignment of the shoulders, hips, knees, and ankles, which necessitates a compensating movement in the hip joint. The head of the femur loses its proper relationship to the other joints and, as a result, experiences extra rotation, grinding into the hip socket like a mortar into a pestle.

In the misaligned hip condition called *coxa valga,* a deformity of the head of the femur increases the angle that the bone inserts into the hip socket, rolling the pelvis forward (top edge) and under (bottom edge). Some medical researchers estimate that walking with this condition results in a load on the hip ten to twenty times greater than the normal load, which is about three times body weight. For a two-hundred-pound man, that means almost five and a half tons— rotating tons—slam into the hip joints. It is my belief that the femur's head is rarely deformed but that the condition is being mimicked by misalignment of the pelvis. With or without an exotic name like *coxa valga,* misalignment in whatever degree opens the door to brutal punishment.

Despite the enormous force it must handle, the synovial sac is more than capable of protecting the hip joint for an hour, a day, a week. But years of pounding and grinding are eventually too much for it. Sooner or later, the cartilage begins scraping away, restricting the joint's range of motion. If the synovium is an air bag, the cartilage is a seat belt. Where two bones meet, this tough, slippery tissue forms a coating and glide surface to prevent direct bone-to-bone contact. Without cartilage, articulation of the joint is impossible because the pain is too excruciating. As the cartilage is gradually being destroyed, the gait-pattern adjusts to use what little cushioning remains, but this adjustment focuses the point pressure of the femur and damages the already-reduced cartilage even more. In addition, pieces of cartilage dislodge and interfere with the finely calibrated ball-and-socket action of the joint, like gravel thrown into the cylinders of an engine as the pistons are pumping up and down.

Modern medicine calls this condition arthritis. It is a disease of unknown origin, we are told. A disease that is incurable. One of the treatments for it is hip replacement. In this procedure, the head of the femur is sawed off, and a new ball and socket is installed, created out of ceramic,

> ## THE ALL-PURPOSE DIAGNOSIS
>
> *Arthritis causes joint deterioration. Thus, all joint deterioration is caused by arthritis.* This clumsy exercise in deduction would earn a failing grade in a freshman college course in logic. Yet in most people over the age of forty, arthritis is routinely blamed for chronic joint pain. Much of this "arthritis" is really symptomatic of musculoskeletal problems and is treatable as such.

metal, and plastic. At the end of five or six hours on the operating table and months of rehabilitation, there's no more synovial fluid or bits of cartilage to get in the way of hip action. The hip feels stronger because it has lost kinesthetic sense. The artificial joint has no nerves. But when the patient gets back on his or her feet, the musculoskeletal demand is ongoing and *unchanged*—that is, still dysfunctional. So the pelvis will still be operating at a dysfunctional angle. It still experiences enormous impact and extra rotation. But the person experiences no pain—at least, not in the new hip joint. Ceramic, metal, and plastic are impervious to pain. The arthritis treatment is a success.

Or is it? Currently, an artificial hip installed in a thirty-year-old man or woman will last about ten years before it breaks down. It must be replaced, which entails another round of *major* surgery and lengthy rehabilitation. With an average life expectancy of eighty years, we can foresee about five hip replacements for that one individual.

Ah, but there's no pain, you may say.

Don't be so sure. The pain shows up in other joints, where it is attributed to spreading arthritis, accidents, overuse, or age. The original muscular pain that accompanied the "bad" hip remains as well. The solution? Well, there's the other hip to replace, as well as knee replacements, diskectomies, spinal fusing, and shoulder reconstruction to be performed. Or the patient may follow the standard advice and give up most forms of "intense" physical activity, to avoid wear and tear on the new joint. They may walk occasionally, or maybe swim. Even so, it becomes harder and harder to get around. The excuses start: *I'm tired. There isn't enough time. My back is bothering me. I couldn't sleep last night.* The body—a machine fueled by motion—is brought to a standstill. All the systems that depend on motion, including digestion, circulation, and respiration, start to starve and go into decline.

Second Thoughts About Hip Replacement Surgery

One day recently, Sean, a top communications executive, sent me his X-rays. He was preparing for hip replacement surgery. He was just back from giving the final pint of blood that he would need for the transfusions that accompany the procedure. He had been reluctantly persuaded to get one more opinion, but his mind was made up. He would go through with it.

Over the phone, I asked him how he felt. "My right hip hurts like hell," he said.

"And that's why you're going to have the operation, right?"

Sean probably thought that was a pretty dumb question. He indicated that the pain was precisely the reason he intended to have the hip replaced.

"In that case, look at your X-rays," I said.

There was a pause while he pulled them out of the envelopes. "Yeah, I am."

"Really look at them. The right one and the left."

Another pause. In an X-ray, cartilage shows up only as a thin shadow. Healthy cartilage is about an eighth of an inch thick. Finally, he said, "Not much cartilage on the right."

"Did anyone ever point out to you that you have even less cartilage in the left hip—the one that doesn't hurt?"

An even longer pause. He could see some cartilage shadow in the right hip, but he had to squint to see it in the left hip.

> ## HIP PAIN
>
> **The muscles aren't replaced when an artificial hip is installed. Yet muscle pain caused much of the agony that was blamed on the "bad" hip. These muscles and the structures they operate are suffering from years of abuse from musculoskeletal dysfunction. Unless that's corrected, they will continue to hurt. Common sense dictates that effective treatment start with working on muscle pain with noninvasive procedures.**

"Uh . . ." Sean, a big-time deal maker, was at a loss for words because he knew what this meant.

If the pain-free left hip had even less cartilage than the right, then the pain in the right hip was not being caused solely by cartilage loss. Some of the pain in the right was attributable to cartilage loss, but some was also attributable to the associated musculature and musculoskeletal mechanisms. Replacing the right hip, in that case, would not cure all the pain but would address only the bone-to-bone component. An even greater potential for bone-to-bone contact existed in the left, yet pain was absent there. Presumably this meant that the musculature in the left hip was in reasonably good condition. Would it be possible to achieve the same outcome in the right without major surgery?

Sean immediately decided to postpone surgery. The body is designed to be bilateral, I explained to him. If the right and left hips could be persuaded to function bilaterally, there is no reason why both couldn't be pain free, since he was already halfway there. And he got there by using the E-cises in this chapter.

In Sean's case, his left hip was rotating and tipped under more than his right, which was also out of position and rotating. The variation in the amount of cartilage was due to the pattern of using that left leg for many years to do more work or play than the right. It doesn't really matter what he was doing, the effect was that the right and left sides were operating on different planes of motion. In other words, they were functioning—dysfunctioning—unilaterally.

As the left side became increasingly unstable, Sean started relying more on the right to walk. However, there was no longer vertical alignment of the load-bearing joints. The right hip tilted under all the more and there was extra rotation grinding away at the cartilage. The pain developed because that was the side Sean had been using the most for the heavy lifting of locomotion (and he no longer had the option to switch sides, since the left was already clapped out). We could see it in his elevated right hip and shoulder. A friendly tailor probably told him at one time that his right leg was longer than the left.

This common misconception shows how far we go to rationalize dysfunction. Both legs are the same length. Only in the rarest of birth defects or childhood accidents is it otherwise. What's happen-

IT'S TOO LATE, I HAVE A NEW HIP

No, it's not too late. If you have had hip replacement surgery and completed your postoperative physical therapy, the E-cises in this chapter are still very useful. Chances are, your hip went "bad" because of musculoskeletal dysfunctions that are still active. You'll need to align your hips and the rest of the load-bearing joints to prevent the symptoms from cropping up elsewhere; otherwise your doctors will soon be talking about replacing the other hip or one of your knees. Also, use the conditioning program in chapter 13.

ing is that the right side is being hoisted up by the muscles and heaved forward and backward to accomplish a semblance of flexion and extension in the leg and hip. Of course, there isn't proper flexion or extension, but rather adduction, abduction, and rotation. The "shorter" left leg is simply showing that the right is dominant and that the pelvis is sloping downward to the left.

Walking on the Surface of the Moon

If you are feeling hip pain, in all probability most of the discomfort is not the direct result of cartilage loss produced by bone-on-bone contact. Deteriorating cartilage tends to pit and crater. Through trial and painful error, the body quickly learns to negotiate this lunar landscape to produce a minimum of suffering. Obeying the muscles, the ball and socket do their best to avoid the worst spots and limit contact with the areas that can't be avoided. Thus, hip movement becomes dependent on an increasingly intricate, restricted, and demanding series of muscular improvisations. For example, the muscles of the low back may get involved in flexing and extending the hip, or trying to. They'll simulate flexion-extension by rotating the hip to avoid the restrictions in the hip socket. This means that instead of riding smoothly front to back, the head of the femur will roll or rock in the socket. The muscles will be taxed beyond their design limits, putting stress on the structures of the low back, while at the same time, cartilage loss will continue to mount, since the gyrating femur is avoiding the worst spots of cartilage loss but is grinding a hole in a new place.

See the vicious circle? The more restricted nondesign movement is used, the less cartilage remains due to devastating point pressure; the less cartilage that remains, the more restricted the nondesign movement and the more devastating the point pressure becomes. The pain closes in from all sides.

But as a measure of just how good the hip joint is at protecting itself, the muscles tend to get to a dysfunctional crisis first. When Sean told me his right hip "hurt like hell," he was only partially correct. His hip ball and socket hurt, but so did the musculature of the lower half of his body. First, the muscles had lost their ability to steer the ball and socket around the bad patches, and bone-to-bone contact resulted. Second, and more important, the musculoskeletal system was showing the wear and tear of years of having to be in the wrong places at the wrong times. As they gave out, the pain increased and the ball-and-socket function declined further.

The site of the pain and the source of the pain don't necessarily coincide: Major hip misalignment leaves its calling card in many different places. It's one reason that physicians tend to have trouble characterizing hip pain. They've persuaded themselves and their patients that hip pain is actually pain in the groin area, or the upper thigh, the knee, or the low back. Their uncertainty leads them to resort to their old friend the X-ray machine. Take a picture of the hip, and behold! Cartilage deterioration.

Since cartilage loss is (incorrectly) regarded as irreversible and since, once it is gone, there seems to be no way to operate the ball and socket without pain (also incorrect), hip replacement becomes a foregone conclusion. But the alternative is to encourage the hips to resume their proper design alignment by reengaging the proper muscles. This is what we'll be doing with the E-cises in this chapter. As we saw in chapter 3, bones do what muscles tell them to do. Reengaging the right muscles will remove the point pressure that's been gouging out the cartilage, relieve the strain and pain on the overstressed muscles and other mechanisms, and return the function of the hip to nearly normal flexion, extension, and rotation. I say "nearly normal" because a certain amount of ball-and-socket management will still be needed due to the preexisting cartilage loss. Even so, the body

---

PRIME MOVERS

Prime movers are muscles that have specific assignments to move specific bones. They work with *synergists,* or muscles that stabilize joints and bones. Because of the central role of the hips, many of both types of muscles *originate* at the pelvic girdle. The other end *inserts* in the bone that is being moved or stabilized. Given the importance of our legs, the prime movers and synergists of the hip are designed to be very powerful.

is capable of providing it as long as its design is intact, particularly if the head of the femur is no longer being repeatedly driven against the unprotected bone structure of the socket.

As for "irreversible" cartilage loss, why of all the tissue in the body would the cartilage be the only one that does not regenerate? The answer is that it does regenerate. Laboratory experiments in Sweden have shown that under the right conditions cartilage, like any tissue, can be grown. Moreover, sports medicine practitioners have long recognized that athletes increase their cartilage density and shock-absorbing capacity during proper training.

Cartilage will regenerate—but only if it is allowed to.

A fractured thighbone, a complete break, will fully mend in about six weeks. But if, during that six weeks, you tried to walk on the leg as if nothing had happened, the injury would never heal properly. Sure, walking with a broken femur is impossible, but so is walking without cartilage. Yet the body tries valiantly to manage it by shifting the point pressure in the hip to healthy cartilage, even as it blasts out crater after crater. Eventually, it has nowhere else to blast. But, since the hip remains misaligned, injured cartilage is never given a chance to regenerate. Then, we try to do what is really impossible: create a hip joint that doesn't need any cartilage at all.

Understanding Hip Flexion and Extension

If there is one silver bullet for treating musculoskeletal disorders, it is the realization that hip misalignment has drastic consequences, from head to toe. (Having said that, I have to add that all load-bearing joint misalignments have drastic consequences.)

In the Egoscue Method program at the clinic, hips are frequently the starting point. Many of the E-cises in this book, no matter what

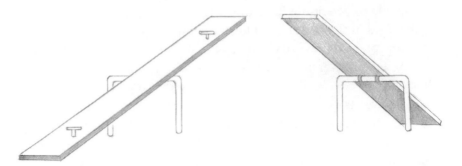

Figure 7–3
Seesaws illustrating hip flexion-extension.

specific joint or pain symptom is being featured, also address hip misalignment. Eliminating hip dysfunction is one of our top priorities simply because of the hips' central role. If the hips are being pushed and pulled out of their proper positions, which is directly under the shoulders and above the knees and ankles, then proper flexion and extension in the torso and lower half of the body are unattainable. This is because of the numerous major muscles, or prime movers, that originate at the pelvis. Weight training to develop shoulder strength, for example, is pointless if the pelvis is out of alignment and the shoulders are drooping forward.

If it is to provide stability, flexibility, and strength in both halves of the body, the pelvic girdle needs a high degree of both latitudinal and longitudinal mobility. It must be able to do at least four things simultaneously. In walking or running, as the right hip extends, the left must flex, and vice versa. Meanwhile, the pelvis has to hold the upper body in a vertical position and at the same time allow for joint rotation to account for terrain variations and other variables.

Get the picture? Don't feel bad if you don't—hip flexion and extension can be hard to imagine. The seesaw example helps:

Flexion and extension require a lot of mobility in the hips, but they also make them vulnerable to dysfunction. (I didn't say fragile or weak.) As strong as they are, the hips, like all bones, must obey the muscles. In a person who sits for hours each day, with his or her body leaning back into the chair with shoulders slumped forward, the muscles are telling the hip to go into flexion. Try it yourself. Sit up straight, with both feet flat on the floor, a distinct arch in your back. Visualize your pelvic girdle as a bowl, with the iliac crests, or hipbones, acting as knobby handles. Put a thumb on each hipbone. Now let your back down and lower it into the rear of the chair. Notice that the hips (and the entire pelvic bowl) move in the same direction by tilting back and down. Meanwhile, the back's arch flattens and then reverses as the top of the spine comes forward, bringing the head and shoulders with it. This is an example of hip flexion.

Clearly your pelvis is obeying your muscles. So is your spine: Hitched to the sacral, a triangular-shaped pedestal attached to the right hip on one side and the left on the other, it's riding atop the pelvic girdle. As the two "handles" move to the rear and down, they tip the sacral pedestal in the same direction. At the same time, the muscles that are anchored to the flexing pelvis and along the spine are tugging downward on the flexible spinal column, shaping it to match the soft concavity of the chairback.

When a functional individual walks or runs, this effect on the spine does not occur because the pelvis maintains a neutral position, alternating from side to side as it flexes and extends. The muscular forces and functions are balanced. They are also *working,* as opposed to disengaged. By contrast, the sitting hip that I've just described has settled back into flexion, where it loses both strength and the ability to readily move back into extension. At the same

THE UPS AND DOWNS OF HIP FLEXION-EXTENSION

Think of two playground seesaws side by side (figure 7-3), both aligned north-south. Looking at them both from the south, the seesaw on the left has its north end up, while the one on the right has its north end down. If the seesaws were running or walking hips (heading south), the left hip would be in extension and the right hip in flexion. The left is tipped forward, the right has moved back. Think of extending imaginary horizontal lines straight out from the hips, front to back, like the seesaws. This seesaw action is precisely what's happening (or should be) when you are walking or running.

HIPS AND CHILDBIRTH

To allow the baby to enter the birth canal, a pregnant woman's hips flare forward and go into extra extension. The design of the female skeleton allows for this (in one of the few musculoskeletal gender differences) by allowing the femur to insert into the hip joint at a greater angle. Even so, women whose hips are locked in flexion, which has become a common characteristic of both sexes, are likely to have trouble during delivery, since the hips are not going to be in the right place. Likewise, a woman with the opposite problem, hips locked in extension, is assuming the birthing position even though the fetus is not ready. This can lead to a premature birth. The E-cises in this chapter help neutralize the hip position, as does the conditioning program in chapter 13.

time, what little upper-body motion occurs has little linkage with the muscular activity (or inactivity) in the pelvis. The back muscles now must keep the spine vertical without the dynamic support of the hips (or the shoulders, which are forward and dropping).

Arthritis and Hip Pain

While some conditions, like heavy cortisone intake and alcoholism, restrict blood circulation to the head of the femur, disease is not the primary cause of hip pain. Even osteoarthritis, which is blamed for so many hip problems, and accidents are secondary factors that occur only after the hip has been put in jeopardy by misalignment.

I have never seen arthritis develop in a joint that was previously active and properly aligned. Never. Given that, as recent clinical tests have shown, moderate regular exercise eases the symptoms of osteoarthritis in the elderly, moderate regular exercise *and* musculoskeletal alignment in younger people would go a long way—if not all the way—toward preventing the onset of the disease in the first place.

Aggressive arthritis—the disease mechanism, not just swelling and cartilage loss—appears to seek out quiet, undisturbed places to set up shop. A joint capsule is a fortress, a world unto itself. Weaken it by blood and oxygen deprivation, which the prioritizing body does to any superficial tissue or systems, and arthritis has the necessary conditions to thrive. If you're feeling hip pain, don't assume that the usual suspects are to blame. Start with the easiest solution first—and see what happens.

E-cises in Response to Hip Pain

Low back, thigh, buttock, and groin pain may originate in your hip—or it may not. But when the rugged hip joint actually starts to hurt, it is a good bet that the muscles and other mechanisms in the region are at least extremely frazzled. No matter where the pain is coming from, these E-cises will help you realign your hip position. The other muscles will appreciate any help they can get.

Given the hips' fundamental role, you may wonder why there are only four E-cises. These ones will alleviate the pain and get the hip into alignment. Once that happens, switch to the conditioning menu in chapter 13 for an ongoing program.

Total time: This menu can take a while because of the Supine Groin Stretch. For severe pain, you may want to do this stretch for forty-five minutes to an hour. For slight pain, fifteen to twenty minutes will do.

Times a day: Once in the morning.

Duration: Do exercises daily until pain abates for twenty-four hours. Once the pain is gone, continue with the menu for one week before switching to the overall conditioning program in chapter 13.

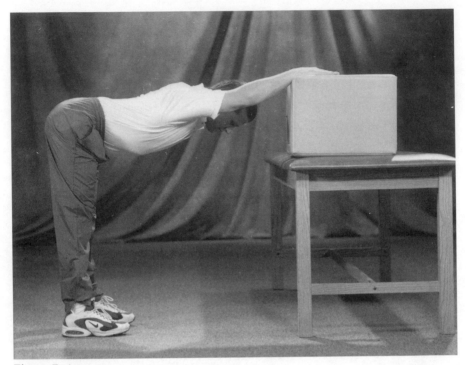

Figure 7–4

- COUNTER STRETCH
  (Figure 7–4)

Place your palms flat on a counter or tabletop that is approximately waist level. (A little higher or lower is okay.) Bend forward at the hips with your arms outstretched on the same plane as your head; your feet, ankles, and knees should be aligned directly under hips. You'll need to inch your feet back to achieve full extension without the hips crimping awkwardly. Let your head fall through your arms, with the hips tilted forward and thighs tight. Hold the position for thirty seconds.

This E-cise takes the hip out of flexion, restores the spine's S-curve, and forces your shoulders to disengage from their compensating position.

• SITTING FLOOR

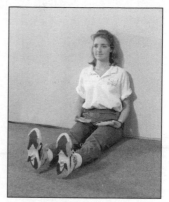

Follow the instructions for Sitting Floor in chapter 6 (figure 6–11, page 95). Concentrate on keeping both feet pulled back evenly.

Sitting Floor works to engage the systems of the lower half of the body with the hip.

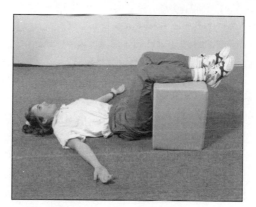

• STATIC BACK

Follow the instructions for Static Back in chapter 5 (figure 5–5, page 70). Take deep breaths. Double-check to ensure that the block is not too high and lifting your low back and hips off the ground.

Static Back uses gravity to put the hips into neutral.

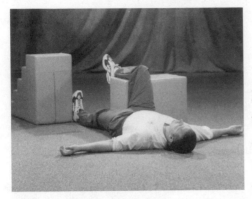

• SUPINE GROIN STRETCH

Follow the instructions for the Supine Groin Stretch in chapter 5 (figure 5–7, page 72). If you use the thigh test to time this one, apply it to get balanced contractions in the right and left thighs.

In this E-cise the groin muscles are pulling on the hips, preventing flexion and extension. This persuades them to let go.

Unfortunately, we have a new national characteristic: Ours has become a nation in hip flexion. Twenty-five years ago, that wasn't the case. Most people had hips that were either functional or in extension (tipped forward). Hip extension is a sign of muscular tightness and strength, and a tight, contracting muscle is one that can be relaxed and readily restored to function. But a muscle that has moved your hips into flexion is weak and tends to stay that way unless a lot of restoration work is done. Even a little restoration would help, but I don't see it happening much outside of my clinic. In fact, the flexion phenomenon is getting worse, and with it an increase in chronic pain and drastic treatment for it. Our magnificent hips can take almost anything but that.

BACKS: CLOSE UP ON THE FAR SIDE

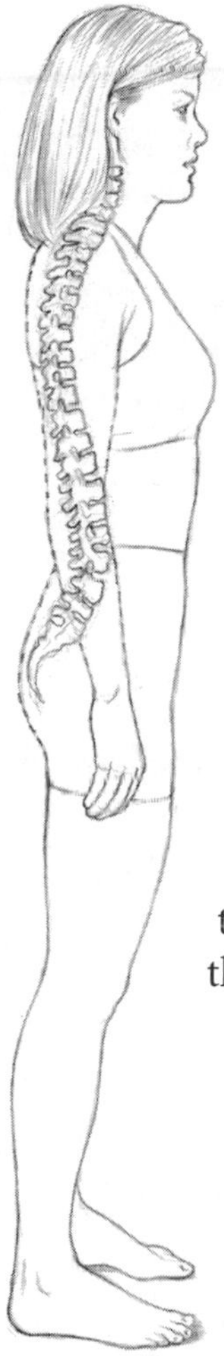

Chronic pain is a traumatic ordeal no matter what its source or symptomatic profile, but chronic back pain has an all-consuming urgency that drives many of us to opt for drastic treatment procedures without stopping for a second thought or opinion. Anyone who has suffered through a severe back spasm knows how excruciating it is. As bad as knee or hip pain can be, back spasms are in a class of their own. The pain chokes off even the inner dialogue that's crucial to an individual's rational decision making. The best time to treat chronic back pain is before it begins or as a spasm moderates, but if you are in the middle of an active back spasm while you are reading these pages, I admire your willpower. It is that power that will allow you to be pain free.

The Importance of Spinal Curves

My job, both on these pages and in the clinic, is to take your mind off your specific back pain symptom. If I succeed in moving you past the pain, we can then go on to address the musculoskeletal dysfunctions that

Figure 8–1

are the real cause of the problem. If not, we will just end up shuffling symptoms around.

When you know why your back is hurting, and only then, you will have the wherewithal to make the pain go away and stay away. The reason, and I'll be quick about saying it, is muscles. That's as succinct as the explanation gets. But a little more information is also necessary. The spine has two anterior curves, lumbar and cervical, basically the low back and the neck. It also has one posterior curve, the thoracic, roughly in the area of the rib cage. This configuration (figure 8–1) exists only because muscles actively work to keep it that way.

Composed of thirty-three individual vertebrae, stacked one atop the other, and threaded through by the spinal cord, the spine—without any muscles—has the characteristics of a thick coral necklace: flexibility without much rigidity. Yet every person uses the spine to hoist into the air a cargo that includes all the major organs, a head with the heft of a bowling ball, and in total, more than half the weight of the human body. We carry that load around as we walk and run, twist and turn, for more than 320,000 waking hours in the first sixty years of life.

In earlier chapters, I referred to the body as an antigravity machine. The drive shaft of that machine is the spine—its unique shape allows us to pull off our extraordinary balancing act. But muscles are also essential, not only to retain the spine's shape but to hold it erect. Conversely, inactive, atrophied, and compensating muscles will alter the lumbar, thoracic, and cervical curves. The muscles that are intended to create and maintain those curves, including the deep paraspinal muscles directly attached to the spine and those of the pelvis and lower half of the body, go on a long sabbatical.

> **Muscular dysfunction tends to occur from the inside out. The deep muscle layers are affected first.**

The muscles around the spine don't all go at once. The rate of atrophy depends on the person's lifestyle and working conditions, but gradually, as the body gets less and less stimulus from the environment, the magical S diminishes, taking with it the spine's flexibility, load-bearing strength, and shock-absorbing capacity.

The Back Has a Last-Resort Mechanism

If you've ever camped out in a tent during a windstorm, you know how important it is to adjust the tent's supporting ropes to allow the outer shell to sway as gusts hit it. There might be a need for more tension to windward and less to leeward. But if the direction of the gale shifts in the night, you'll have to climb out of your warm

> **Muscles that do not move are soon muscles that cannot move.**

sleeping bag and make changes, otherwise the tent will shake and flap. The musculature of the torso, as we move, is doing the same thing on a nanosecond-by-nanosecond basis. The muscles that adjust the position of the spine maintain a constant dynamic interaction to keep it upright and fully functional.

The arrangement is flawless, except in one respect: Muscles only follow orders. If they are not being told to move, they stay right where they are. When they aren't moving enough, then the entire back, as happens with other subsystems of our musculoskeletal system, isn't moving nearly enough.

Abandoned by the muscles, and losing the integrity of its curves, the spine is at the mercy of gravity—and gravity is merciless: What goes up must come down. Without the flexibility that allows for balance, rigidity sets in. Confronted with an unstable spine, the body has one last-resort mechanism for utilizing what little power remains in atrophying muscles: It throws them into contraction. The contracting muscles, however, cannot defeat gravity by holding the spine in place by sheer strength alone; the spine has too many moving parts. And since the upper torso is designed to flex forward, the muscles grudgingly allow flexion, until the structure of the spine reaches its limits and freezes in place.

BEDTIME

With a severe active back spasm, it may be necessary, as a first step, to spend a day or two in bed to allow the pain to subside enough for E-cise therapy to begin. Bed rest will limit the muscular demands that are moving the disk or bone into contact with nerves. But when the pain eases, don't go back to business as usual. Use this "window" of pain relief to begin therapy. And please don't stay in bed more than a couple of days; it doesn't take long for important functions to begin deteriorating from inactivity.

To get a clearer picture of this sequence, pack up the tent, climb into your 4 × 4 and head for home. The windstorm has changed to a blizzard, the road is icy, and a deer jumps out of the woods in front of the truck. You hit the brakes, and they lock. That's what's happening with the muscles. Back in the careening truck, you swing the steering wheel to the right and left, trying to prevent a skid. The truck fishtails wildly. With back pain, the major compensating muscles, like a steering wheel, yank on the spine in a desperate attempt to keep it semimobile and reasonably upright. But the spine can't win under those circumstances. Short of total paralysis and rigor mortis, there is no escaping from motion: The body must move. But as the dysfunctional body moves, even a little, it wrings out the bones, muscles, ligaments, tendons, and cartilage of the torso.

The solution to back pain is based on a pure cause-and-effect connection: Go after the muscles, not the spine. While some back pain is caused by damage to the spine or its components—a herniated disk, nerve impingement, or other conditions—most active back pain is the result of ongoing muscular action (and/or inaction). Put a stop to that dysfunctional, nondesign muscular activity, and the pain will subside. I have seen it happen literally thousands of times.

Treating the Herniated Disk

At the clinic, we see more clients with herniated disks than with any other back pain symptom. Many of them bring X-rays that show that the disk—a tough pad of tissue that acts as a cushion between vertebrae—has been squeezed by the bones until it comes into contact with a nerve. The disk is either bulging like a balloon that's being squeezed, or it actually ruptures, with its softer inner core material oozing out like a jelly doughnut leaking its filling. I look at the pictures and say, "Yes, that's definitely a herniated disk."

"The doctor wants to surgically remove the piece that's pressing on the nerve."

I nod and ask, "Don't you think your back was designed to use all of that disk?"

"But it's against the nerve."

"Why? How did it get there?" And since by that point we've discussed some of the basics of human biomechanics, I usually get this response:

"Muscles put it there."

"Right. And muscles can take it out of there."

There are five E-cises that are effective for mitigating musculoskeletal pain in the low back.

> **Total time: Twenty minutes.**
>
> **Times a day: Once in the morning.**
>
> **Duration: Do the exercises daily until pain abates for forty-eight hours, and then continue the menu for ten days before switching to the overall conditioning program in chapter 13. Don't be impatient. If your back has been hurting twenty-four hours a day, initial pain relief of an hour or two indicates progress. If you seem to be plateauing, increase the repetitions.**

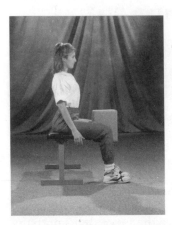

• SITTING KNEE PILLOW SQUEEZES

This E-cise was introduced in chapter 6 (figure 6–10, page 94). Follow the instructions there, and make sure you sit right on the edge of the bench. Keep your feet flat on the floor, hip-width apart, toes pointing straight ahead. Do three sets of fifteen. Do the squeezes slowly and evenly on both sides.

This E-cise strengthens the hip's abductor/adductors to help pull the back out of flexion.

• STATIC BACK KNEE PILLOW SQUEEZES
  (Figure 8–2)

Get into the Static Back position in chapter 5 (figure 5–5, page 70), and place a pillow between the knees. Using the inner thighs,

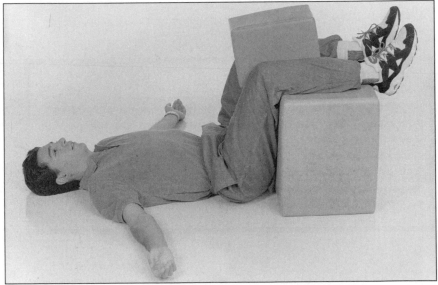

Figure 8–2

squeeze the pillow and release evenly. The feet remain parallel to each other. Relax your stomach. Do three sets of fifteen.

This E-cise allies the adductor/abductors with the force of gravity and disengages the lower extremities.

- MODIFIED FLOOR BLOCK
  (Figure 8–3)

Lie on your stomach with your forehead on the floor. Your feet should be pigeon-toed and the buttocks relaxed. Rest your elbows on blocks so that the arms and hands are in the "Don't shoot, sheriff—I give up" position. Make sure your shoulders are level from right to left. Breathe deeply, and relax the upper body. Don't press your arms into the blocks; let the chest and stomach fall into the floor, and that will cause the hips to tilt forward. Hold the position for six minutes. This E-cise disengages the shoulders.

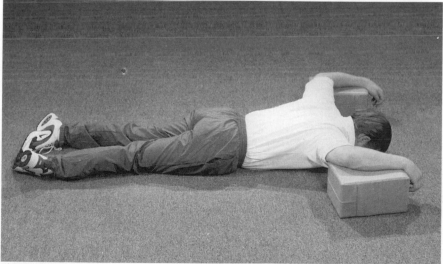

Figure 8–3

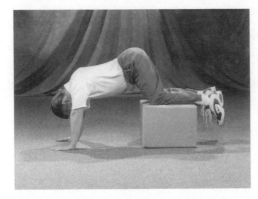

• STATIC EXTENSION
  (POSITION)

See chapter 4 (figure 4–7, page 56) for instructions on Static Extension, but make one important change: Do the E-cise on the floor rather than using a block for elevation. Don't let Static Extension spook you: Generally, extreme flexion causes a herniated disk, and this E-cise promotes, as the name implies, extension, relieving the pressure on the disk. Make sure you come forward onto your hands so that the hips move in front of the knees. This will allow the back to sway and restore the missing lumbar arch. It helps to have someone watch to verify that your back is swaying and not flat— or worse, rounding. Your stomach muscles should be totally slack. Be assured that the body won't let you aggravate the herniation; pain would immediately short-circuit the procedure. Hold the position for one minute.

• AIR BENCH

See chapter 4 (figure 4–8, page 57) for instructions on Air Bench. Keep your shoulders and head against the wall throughout. Hold for one to two minutes.

This E-cise relinks the ankles, knees, and hips.

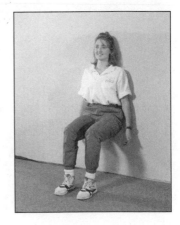

When the pain subsides, which should occur after a week of doing the above routine, add the following E-cises:

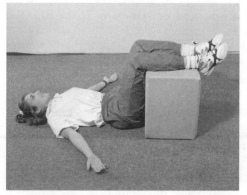

• STATIC BACK

The instructions for Static Back are in chapter 5 (figure 5–5, page 70). Don't overdo this one: After an hour it has diminishing returns. I know it feels good, but it's counterproductive to spend all morning or afternoon in Static Back. Inactivity will take a toll. Hold for only five to ten minutes. Static Back uses gravity to get the structures back on the same plane, but they also must have vertical loading.

• SUPINE GROIN STRETCH

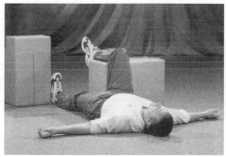

The instructions for Supine Groin Stretch are also in chapter 5 (figure 5–7, page 72). The problem here is underdoing it. Give the E-cise plenty of time to work. Hold for at least ten minutes per side. The groin muscles are powerful, and it takes time to persuade them to let go.

• AIR BENCH (SECOND SET)

See the first set of E-cises on the previous page.

THE NEED TO KNOW BEFORE SURGERY

Removal of the lumbar disks or pieces of them has become a common surgical procedure. If you are considering it, first ask the doctors four questions:

1. Why is the disk herniated?
2. Don't I need the portion of the disk you'll remove?
3. Will I be able to resume all my previous physical activities?
4. Will this problem recur with another disk?

Be skeptical if you're told, in answer to the first question, that the damage to the disk is related to your age or an accident. As for the second, your back was designed to use each disk—all of each disk. The question about physical activity is important because treatment that purports to cure should restore your health and functions, not curtail them. Finally, a recurrence is likely after surgery because the musculoskeletal problems that caused the first herniation will still be at work.

If the pain continues undiminished, drop the first five E-cises and do only the three additional ones (Static Back, Supine Groin Stretch, and Air Bench); the lingering pain is telling us that we must first remove the extra rotation from your hips. After about a week, try including the first five items, adding one or two at a time every couple of days. Let common sense be your guide. Back pain is a symptom of conditions that have been developing for years. It will take more than a few minutes to get results, and some of the E-cises, since they work on different muscles and functions, may take longer than others.

Spine Tuning

Although most low back pain is directly related to changes in the spine's curvature, pain isn't a structural problem; nor is it permanent. You can feel how muscles sculpt your own back by sitting on the edge of a desk chair. Keep your feet flat on the floor, hip-width apart. Lean to the rear until the back feels like it's vertical. Relax your stomach muscles and shoulders. Now, reach around with your right or left hand and place it on the small of the back just above the waist.

What do you feel? If you're like most people, the answer is, "Nothing much—a back." But you should notice immediately a pronounced concavity or arch—the lumbar curve. There's no missing it when it's there. If you have any doubt, it's not there (figure 8–4).

Keep your hand on the small of your back. Slowly pull your head back and your shoulders together without tightening the stomach muscles, but do create some tension in the shoulder blades and the upper back area. Notice a change? There should be even more of a lumbar arch. And you probably experienced some hip movement (rotating forward) in the process. Now settle back into a natural position. You'll feel the arch straighten and disappear while the head sinks and shoulders round forward.

As this happens, the lumbar spine moves to the posterior along with the hips. The low back is going into flexion. It is seeking to jackknife, to fold forward at the waist. Extension—the ability to bring the spine into a full upright posture with the head centered over the pelvis—is compromised. The fulcrum point of vertebral leverage, meanwhile, shifts in the opposite direction (figure 8–5).

Starting to get complicated, isn't it? Visualize vertebral leverage like this: Suppose that between each vertebra there is a small, perfectly round marble. (There

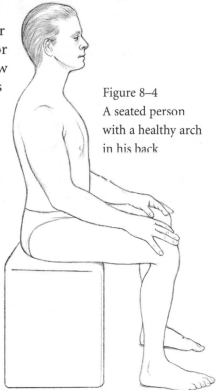

Figure 8–4
A seated person
with a healthy arch
in his back

isn't, we're just supposing.) In a functional back, the marble is right in the center. The vertebrae twist and turn smoothly, the edges ascend and descend (figure 8–6). But in flexion, the marble is forced toward the rear of the body, so that attempts to extend or straighten the spine are no longer borne by the entire vertebral disk; worse, the altered fulcrum point—the marble—means that the levers formed by the surfaces of the vertebrae are rising and falling with increased force on the posterior edge of the disk (figure 8–7). This intense point pressure squashes the disk and eventually causes it to begin bulging or extruding material.

> ## WHEN CHRONIC BACK PAIN DOESN'T HURT
>
> **Pain is a symptom, and so is numbness. If one or both of your legs is numb, the condition may be evidence of major nerve impingement by a disk or lumbar structure. Don't procrastinate. An MRI will show you what's going on. Then work with your health advisers to develop a treatment plan that recognizes that the problem was caused by muscular dysfunction.**

Flexion is also hard on the facet joints of the spine, which form the interconnections between vertebrae. With enough flexion, the spine loses its marbles altogether, and the facets end up as the fulcrum points. This is double trouble. First, the facets start breaking down, since they have little shock-absorbing capacity and range of motion. Second, the posterior edge of the disk is caught in the jaws of a powerful vise that is being cranked another turn every time the individual moves his or her back.

The E-cises that I recommend are designed to keep the "marbles" in the center between individual vertebrae. The idea is to release the pressure on the disk enough either to allow its natural elasticity to retract the extruded material off the nerve, or to pull that entire vertebral component toward the rear and give the nerve back its space. If the facet joints are also involved, they'll get relief simultaneously.

Contracting muscles complicate the process, since they really don't want to let go. I can't blame them. In an ultimate sense, the

choice between permanent contraction and permanent relaxation
is a choice between life and death.
Muscles have a tendency to
hang on to the contraction as
long as possible. With low
back pain, muscle relaxants
can be of some help because
they force the muscles to relax and stop pressing the
bone or disk into the nerve.

Limited bed rest can have
the same effect by removing
the stimulus. Let's use George
as an example. He has a habit
of bending down to tie his
shoes in the morning. George
doesn't do it when he's lying
flat on his back in agony from
low back pain. But once the
pain is gone for a few days,
he'll resume his shoe-tying
routine, and those muscles
will again be receiving or-

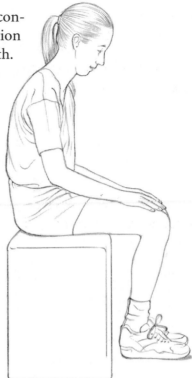

Figure 8–5
A seated person with hips and back in
flexion.

ders to contract. Likewise, with relaxant drugs, the muscles will return to their old ways once the treatment ends. A person who
continues to take muscle relaxants will be too lethargic to move
enough to trigger another episode of pain.

This pattern of behavior modification, it should be noted, explains why recent studies have shown that people with episodes of
severe back pain who seek treatment from doctors, physical therapists, or chiropractors have about the same recovery rates as those
who do not. In both circumstances, the stimulus is being changed.
The do-nothing group "takes it easy" and through trial and error
learns how to avoid movement that causes pain. In short, their self-
treatment is to restrict motion. Those who undergo surgical, therapeutic, and manipulative procedures are doing basically the same

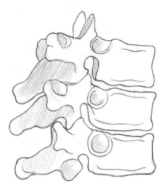

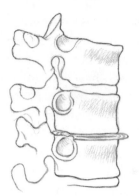

Figure 8–6
The vertebrae shown in
relation to each other.

Figure 8–7
A vertebral disk under
pressure.

thing. The body is actually curing itself by finding a new way around
the pain. The problem is that the body eventually runs out of painless alternative routes.

Road Signs:
Danger—Sharp Thoracic Curve Ahead

Let's catch up with George, now that he's out of bed, and travel with
him a little way. He teaches himself to tie his shoes using the thoracic back, the spine's major posterior curve (with convexity to the
rear). The thoracic back is pulled forward and down by gravity since
it is designed to accommodate forward flexion. As a result, it has
more range of motion in that direction, and as the lumbar and cervical curves approach their limits, the thoracic curve keeps going—
to a point. George quickly learns to use it to replace his lost
functions. For instance, to tie his shoes, he sits down and brings his
right foot up to the top of his left knee. He bends forward until his
lower back freezes and then, to reach the laces, flexes the rest of the
way with his thoracic back. Try this yourself: Sit in a desk chair with
your hips all the way to the rear. Let the back settle down. Now reach
for the phone, keeping your back and hips stationary. Notice that
the upper back and shoulders handle the flexion demand. Many

people spend hours at a time in that position. Like George, they substitute the thoracic back for low back functions.

It's a trade-off, one that has a substantial price. When the thoracic back is in flexion, pulling forward on the skeletal components of the upper torso, the opposing muscles of extension, rotation, and lateral movement tighten in reaction. This leads to a restriction of motion in the upper back and shoulders. In addition, the body is somewhat top-heavy to begin with, and now gravity gets even more traction; the shoulders continue to round forward, and the head droops all the more. What's next? More thoracic flexion, more tightness, more of everything except function.

Thereafter thoracic back pain tends to disguise itself. The tightness gives way to burning in the area between the shoulder blades, the neck gets stiff, and turning the head from side to side or up and down becomes difficult or painful. Another common symptom is numbness in the shoulders, arms, and hands while sleeping or resting in a chair. What's happening is that the joints of the upper torso are being pulled out of alignment, constricting the circulation and creating extra friction.

> ### STOMACH TROUBLE
>
> **Everybody wants a flat stomach, but the worst way to get one is to deliberately contract your abdominal muscles. This holds your hips and spine in flexion, preventing them from achieving neutral positions. Healthy abdominals are intended to work as back stabilizers, not prime movers. Relax your abdominals and flatten them with diet and exercise.**

Head position is a real thoracic-back-problem indicator. Taylor, a client in his late fifties, discovered that it had been years since he had raised his head to look straight out. His line of sight angled downward to a point about ten feet in front of his feet. To look at the horizon, he had to lean back at the hips. Thoracic back flexion had thrust his shoulders and head so far forward that it was impossible for him to look up at the sky without lying flat on his back. When I'm out driving, I often see people just like Taylor, whose thoracic back restrictions prevent them from reacting to what's ahead beyond a car length or two. Moreover, many drivers—and I mean *many* as in millions—can't move their heads easily to the left and right to look over their shoulders before making lane changes. I'm afraid that even side and rearview mirrors are falling outside the comfortable range of motion for many drivers.

Unfortunately, even if the highway patrol started pulling people over and giving them range-of-motion tests, it wouldn't do much good. Thoracic back dysfunctions tend to get diagnosed as rotator cuff, shoulder, and neck problems. Those conditions, however, are only symptoms, and treating them would make the roads only temporarily safer. For a few months, Taylor and his like wouldn't be such menaces, but soon the effects of the corrective surgery or therapy would diminish. Tunnel vision would return. Structures—including the structures of the back—do not break down without a powerful reason.

Once I see rounded shoulders and hear about tightness in the middle of the back, I usually don't need to look any further for the cause. A client who tells me that they have a feeling of tightness in their upper back usually gives me their very next message in body language: They shrug and waggle their shoulders, a classic effort to loosen up tight muscles. It doesn't work, though. I suggest that instead they stand up straight with their shoulders back and toes pointed in (pigeon-toed). Immediately the tightness eases. Why? It seems counterintuitive, since in terms of anatomical geography the toes and shoulders don't even share the same hemisphere. But it works because the pigeon-toed stance brings the pelvis back in line with the shoulders. Upper back tightness is telling us that the shoulders are hanging in midair without structural support from the load-bearing joints or interaction with the musculature of the pelvic girdle.

These six E-cises will relieve thoracic back symptoms by reuniting and realigning the two halves of the body.

> **Total time: This menu can take a while because of the Supine Groin Stretch. For severe pain, you may want to do this stretch for forty-five minutes to an hour. For slight pain, fifteen to twenty minutes will do.**
> **Times a day: Once in the morning.**

> **Duration:** Do the exercises daily until pain abates for forty-eight hours, and then continue the menu for ten days before switching to the overall conditioning program in chapter 13. Don't be impatient. If your back has been hurting twenty-four hours a day, initial pain relief of an hour or two indicates progress. If you seem to be plateauing, increase the repetitions.

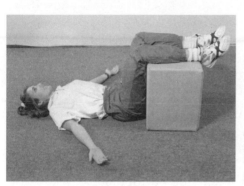

• STATIC BACK

The instructions for Static Back can be found in chapter 5 (figure 5–5, page 70).

• REVERSE PRESSES
(Figure 8–8)

Assume the Static Back position, with legs propped and knees bent at ninety degrees. Place your elbows straight out from your shoulders, bend your elbows, form loose fists with each hand, and

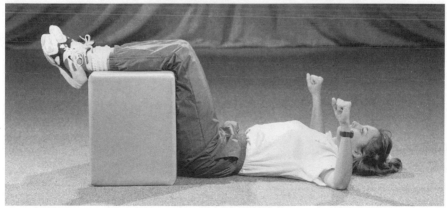

Figure 8–8

point the knuckles up toward the ceiling. Squeeze the shoulder blades together by pressing the elbows straight down into the floor. Don't jerk. Concentrate on the shoulder blades coming together. You are getting them out of the forward position this way. Hold for a moment and release. Repeat fifteen times.

- PULLOVERS
  (Figure 8–9 a and b)

While in the Static Back position, clasp your hands together tightly, and extend your elbows straight toward the ceiling (a). Continuing to hold both arms straight, bring them back behind your head, either to the floor or as far as they will go without bending (b). Then return to the starting position. Relax your abdominal muscles, and don't rush. Repeat fifteen times. This E-cise reminds the ball and socket that it is not exclusively a hinge.

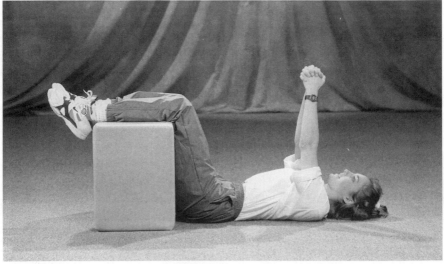

Figure 8–9a

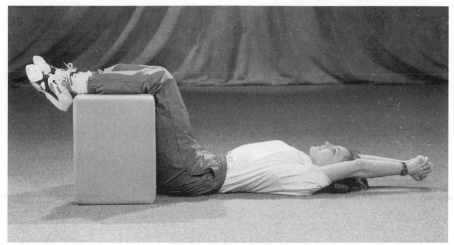

Figure 8–9b

- **FLOOR BLOCK**
  (Figure 8–10 a, b, and c)

This E-cise, done in three positions, runs the ball-and-socket functions of the arm and shoulder joints through their full range of motion.

Figure 8–10a

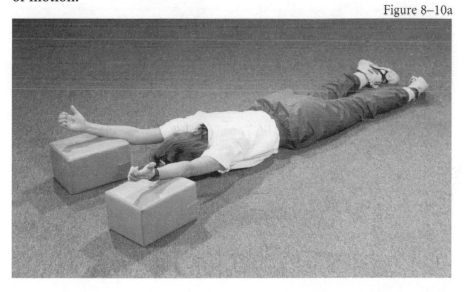

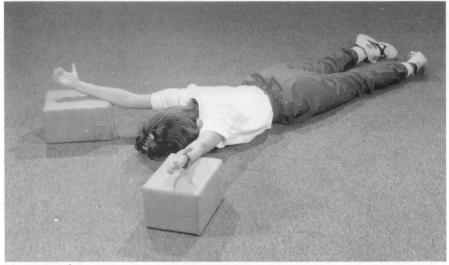

Figure 8–10b

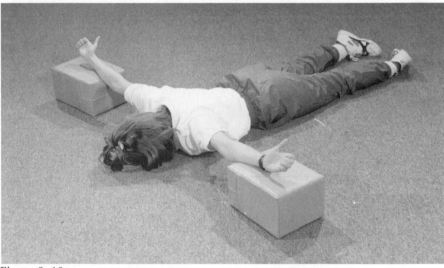

Figure 8–10c

One: Lie on your stomach, face-down, arms over your head, with elbows straight and feet pigeon-toed (a). Rest your arms (at the wrists) on six-inch blocks, making light fists with the hands (don't clench them tightly) and pointing the thumbs toward the ceiling. Rotate your arms into this position from the shoulders, not from the elbows. Place your forehead on the floor, and keep the neck, shoulders, buttocks, and stomach relaxed. Let your hips fall forward into the ground. Hold this first position for one minute.

Two: Remain lying on your stomach with your body in the same position (b). Slide your arms—with the blocks—to forty-five-degree angles. Remember to keep your neck, shoulders, buttocks, and stomach relaxed. As in position one, your arms must rotate at the shoulders to bring the thumbs around to point at the ceiling. Hold for one minute.

Three: Remain lying on your stomach with the body in the same position (c). Slide your arms—with the blocks—to ninety-degree angles. Keep your neck, shoulders, buttocks, and stomach relaxed. Rotate your arms at the shoulders. Hold for one minute.

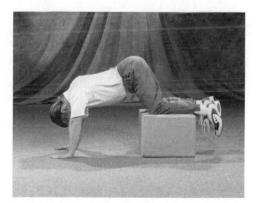

• STATIC EXTENSION

The instructions for Static Extension are in chapter 4 (figure 4–7, page 56). This E-cise reforges the links from head to hip.

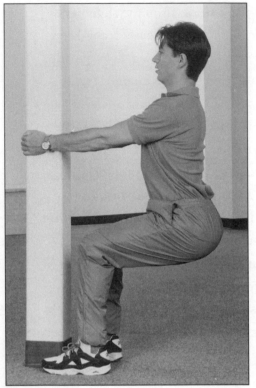

Figure 8–11

- SQUAT
  (Figure 8–11)

Holding on to a rail, pole, or doorknob for support, bend your knees and arch your lower back. Keep your torso straight. Lower your body so that the knees and hips are parallel. The arms should be straight and the knees aligned with hips and feet. The torso remains vertical throughout. Hold for one to two minutes.

This E-cise works the proper lower-body muscles and structures to accomplish movement, while the top is under proper vertical load.

How about the cervical curve? I've mentioned it in passing, but symptoms of cervical back dysfunctions (like lumbar and thoracic dysfunctions) show up in the neck. Actually, the cervical curve is the neck, in that its seven vertebrae extend from the shoulder girdles to the base of the skull. I'll give it detailed treatment in chapter 11.

Five "Frictional" Characters and One Plot Structure

A few pages back, I made this flat statement: "Pain isn't a structural problem." When I wrote that, I knew I was leaving myself open for someone to say, "What about spinal stenosis, spondylolisthesis, spondylolysis, spondylosis, and scoliosis?" The answer is that those conditions are also muscular.

The first four—stenosis, spondylolisthesis, spondylolysis, and spondylosis—are needlessly daunting terms. Usually stenosis involves the formation of calcium deposits as a result of friction caused by musculoskeletal misalignment. The body always reacts to friction. It has to, otherwise vital components will be worn away. The bones' defensive mechanism against friction is to generate an extra layer or blob of calcium. But this solution is not ideal since the calcium interferes with the movement of the vertebrae. Given enough friction and enough calcium, the process creates nerve impingement. The standard surgical remedy is to remove the lamina of the vertebrae—basically, one slope of the arch or ridge that runs along the posterior of the spine—enter the canal, and scrape away the calcium.

I have rarely seen a case of stenosis where this procedure was really necessary. Yes, there is calcium in the spinal canal, and there is nerve impingement. But if the lumbar, thoracic, and cervical curves are restored to a functional state, the spinal cord and the branching nerve roots usually have enough room to operate without interference.

Likewise, spondylolisthesis, spondylolysis, and spondylosis can be treated in the same way. In spondylolisthesis, a shifting of vertebrae narrows the spinal canal. Spondylolysis is the degeneration and fusion of the articulating part of a vertebra; spondylosis deals with lesions of the spine. All these conditions occur because of muscular dysfunction, as weak and compensating muscles allow the structure of the spine to be displaced and damaged.

A slightly different phenomenon occurs with scoliosis. But even so, it too is muscular and not structural. It most often affects adolescents who are experiencing sudden growth spurts. At puberty the muscles and their functions may have a difficult time keeping up with the burgeoning skeletal structure, particularly when the young person changes his or her established patterns of behavior, which is exactly what those entering their teenage years tend to do. Scoliosis affects girls more than boys primarily because girls' physicality can go through a more abrupt transition. The two extreme possibilities are that a so-called "tomboy" becomes a proper "young lady," and a girl who has shown little interest in the rough-and-tumble of sports suddenly discovers her athletic talent. In both instances, coinciding with the growth spurt is a drastic modification in the demand that's being put on the musculoskeletal system.

RIGHTIES AND LEFTIES

The effect of being either right-handed or left-handed comes primarily in the context of less developed functions on the side that is not dominant. In a motion-rich environment, this isn't a problem; there is enough stimulus on both sides. Since we are all motion-deprived these days, never exercise a right-side function without giving equal treatment to the left (and vice versa).

Teenagers go from books to basketball in a flash, or from monkey bars to mascara. These changes take the body by surprise, with the result that the body forgets about being bilateral. Adolescent boys, I should add, generally—though not always—make a more gradual transition from their prepuberty behavior patterns. Hence, their bilateral functions are less threatened. The spine of a girl (or boy) diagnosed with scoliosis is under extreme pressure, however. Various functions—some newly strengthened, others weakening from disuse—are pulling on it (or offering inadequate opposing resistance) to such an extent that the spine begins to curve laterally.

Scoliosis can be treated with a program of balanced muscular stimulation. In the clinic, we remind the body that it is a bilateral machine. What happens on the right side must also take place on the left. In this and every circumstance that the body confronts, the old architectural slogan is absolutely right: Form follows function. Reintroduce proper design function, and the form—the structure—isn't a problem. Back pain, no matter what it is called, is most often a symptom of a breakdown of form that has been generated by a loss of function. The precipitating event can be hormones or happenstance: a new job, a change in physical routine, or an illness, perhaps. Whatever the contributing factors, a pain treatment that starts with function will rarely require you to go after the body's form.

CHAPTER 9

SHOULDERS: LOCKED IN THE BOX

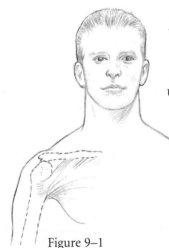

Figure 9–1

Your purse weighs a ton. Or your old slam-dunk isn't what it used to be. Perhaps it's because your shoulders aren't what they used to be. The pages ahead deal with a painful anatomical disappearing act that threatens to change the very definition of what it is to be human.

Darwin in Reverse

If I was to name the one musculoskeletal component that is undergoing the most serious devolution, it would be the shoulders. We don't use them much these days. Our world of motion has been squeezed into an invisible three-by-four-foot box that hangs in midair directly in front of us, covering an area roughly from the midthighs to the armpits. We reach into it to answer the phone, adjust the TV, and unlock the car door. We do little else outside this box; we take it with us wherever we go.

Equipped with this invisible template that guides modern motion, we have simply forgotten to routinely use more than fifty percent of the shoulder's functions. As a result, when a task comes along that the shoulder is designed to do but that is outside the box, we start hurting. Paint the house? Wrestle a suitcase out of the overhead cargo bin in an airplane? Prune the apple tree? Rake leaves? Hit a tennis ball? These jobs are no big deal—we have the muscles, joints, and bones to do all of them *easily* and safely. What we're lacking is a fully functional range of motion, a capability that we were born with and developed as young children, but then lost, not because of age but because we started restricting our motion to the box and have done so for years. We left our shoulder functions outside, like tricycles, roller skates, and pogo sticks abandoned in the grass of the front yard to rust away. Shoulder pain is the price exacted for our neglect of them.

Time-lapse photography would show that the box is getting smaller as the head comes forward, the shoulders round forward, and the spine takes on the shape of a C (figure 9–2). In the final configuration some of the muscles are shut down completely, while others are attempting to move joints that have been nearly immobilized by friction and biomechanical restrictions. Under these conditions episodic shoulder pain is a warning: Don't push the limits, stay in the box! And chronic shoulder pain tells us that the steadily shrinking box has now become too small to accommodate even the most limited, routine movement. "I should have known better . . ." is an all-purpose lament that doctors, therapists, and chiropractors hear every day. Fill in the blank with ". . . than to have carried both my laptop and my suitcase on the trip," or ". . . than to have played thirty-six holes of golf last Saturday." The next line is always, "And now my shoulder is killing me." Out of all the varied pain symptoms of musculoskeletal dysfunction, shoulder pain seems to come as the biggest surprise. It's as if we expect our backs, hips, and knees to hurt from time to time, but not our shoulders. There are two explanations for our surprise: One, the shoulders are efficient at painlessly using a steadily dwindling range of motion, ingeniously supported by modern technology. Two, shoulder pain produces deep anxiety because it seems to directly threaten our survival. Much of this attitude comes from where we are today and how we got here.

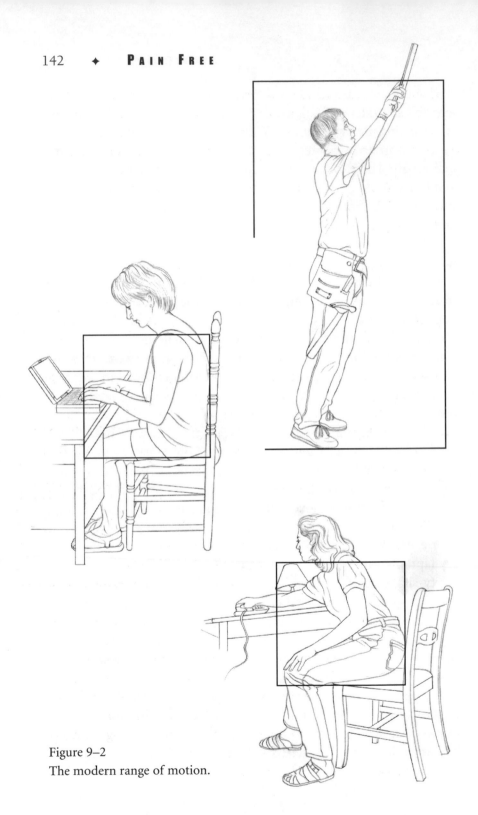

Figure 9–2
The modern range of motion.

Primitive hunters and gatherers depended on their feet and legs as vehicles to deliver edible objects to powerful jaws and sharp teeth. Lunch was served only to those who could catch it. When farmers, warriors, and artisans emerged, however, they used their hands to accomplish complicated work. As humans developed from creatures that ate with their feet to creatures that eat with their hands, shoulder function became even more essential. Shoulders and upper limbs emerged as equal partners with the legs and feet.

Our transformation was a small step and, literally, a great stretch of the shoulders.

The refinement of shoulder function went on from there to carrying (children and supplies), throwing (weapons), and manipulating (tools). Without functional shoulders these things cannot happen.

Few people suspect that the tightness or pain might have something to do with the fact that before their encounter with the paintbrush, the golf club, or the suitcase, they had not been outside the box in months or even years. They'd been trapped there without lifting their arms above their heads, without pulling or pushing, and without swinging, flexing, or fully extending their arms.

When they get to the doctor's office, however, they do ask, "What's wrong with my shoulder?" The usual answer they get is tendinitis. The *-itis* diseases are rampant these days. Technically, *-itis* is a suffix that can be attached to any noun: *catitis*, for example. What does it mean? Not much more than "catlike," denoting similarity. However, at some point *-itis* started being used to denote inflammation, and that is the meaning that we are stuck with today; a fancy suffix that means less than it implies when pinned onto a noun. A doctor who says you have tendinitis isn't making a diagnosis as much as offering a vague observation; namely, that you have swelling and pain.

As you can probably tell, I'm impatient with this word *tendini-*

> ### LIVING HAND TO MOUTH
>
> **Many anthropologists believe the development of key human social characteristics started when we brought food to our mouths rather than our mouths to the food.**

WHEN WAS THE LAST TIME YOU . . .

Got down on the floor?

Hung by your hands?

Crawled on your hands and knees?

Threw a ball overhand?

Threw a ball underhand?

Climbed a tree?

Bore weight over your head?

Reached behind you, left and right?

Whirled your arms at the shoulder sockets?

Shoveled?

Climbed over a fence?

Climbed under a fence?

Stretched on tiptoes?

Raked leaves or grass clippings?

Pushed a heavy object?

Pulled a heavy object?

Swung a bat with both hands?

Swung a stick or a racket with one hand?

Carried more than ten pounds in each hand?

Lifted more than twenty pounds with both hands off the floor?

Delivered a forceful blow with your arm and hand?

Held both arms up and out to the sides?

Put both your hands on top of your head?

Balanced on one foot?

Balanced on one foot while off the ground (atop a stump, stool, or bench)?

Walked up a flight of stairs?

Took more than one step at a time (ascending and descending)?

Danced?

tis. I don't like the suggestion that shoulder or joint pain is a disease, something a person catches like the flu or TB, or is predisposed to genetically, or comes down with by accident. Pain and swelling in the shoulder are symptoms of musculoskeletal misalignment. They are symptoms of living inside the box. See for yourself how much time you spend there. Make a list of your routine activities: typing, reading, driving, and so on. Note the ones that are carried out in the box and those done outside. The former will probably predominate. Deliberately climb out of the box, and see how long you can remain at large. Time yourself. Most "productive" activity is done inside the box. To escape for any length of time, you'll find it necessary to have a life that allows you to dance, shadow-box, fool around, and generally act "childlike."

If you go through the list and answer each question directly—not with "It's been a while" but with the actual length of time—I think you'll be shocked. There will be some activities that you haven't done in years, and not because they are difficult, dangerous, or physically taxing. Few people reach directly over their heads more than a couple of times a year, let alone bear any weight in that position. Yet all of us have a carefully calibrated mechanism for doing that. What happens to the mechanism when we don't use it? The function is lost.

> ### THE FORGOTTEN JOINT
>
> **Modern motion is so limited and is based so much on repeated patterns that we have eliminated the shoulders from most routine activities. We assume our shoulders are working fine—because they're not working much at all. It comes as a shock when we ask the shoulders to do something simple and get pain instead.**

That may not seem like such a big deal. After all, if I don't need to extend my arms over my head, there's no point to my having that function—is there?

Reaching into the box during the course of both work and play, shrugging the shoulders, and hitting a golf ball—no matter how repetitively or energetically—are not sufficient to keep functional the muscles by which we reach toward the sky. If those muscles become dysfunctional, then the posture muscles involved in holding our shoulders back, heads up, and spines in the S-curve are also prevented from doing their job. Inactivity disables both sets of muscles. The entire unit breaks down. The same goes for each of the activities on my list: The muscles that are needed to throw a ball properly, hold the arms outstretched to the right and left, push a heavy object, and so on, are all members of the same team. If any of them doesn't show up, the rest are left to play a losing game.

The list is an excellent diagnostic tool because it is not composed of "some can—some can't" items. All of us "can" perform each of those activities—the human body comes equipped with the capability for them—but few of us do. Whatever reason we may offer—ranging from "it's undignified" to "I don't feel like it,"—by way of explanation, if we don't get down on the floor, balance on one leg, or climb over a fence, it needs to be examined for what it really is: a symptom of ill health. Musculoskeletal functions that are not regularly used become inaccessible. Thus, the result is devastatingly simple: Those who can, do; those who can't, don't. Ability has nothing to do with coordination, athletic skill, or strength. The sole requirement is function. We end up living in the box because we cannot live pain free outside it.

> ## MORE THAN MUSCLES
>
> **Kinesthetic sense is not limited to muscles. It involves all the other systems and subsystems of the body. The lymph system, for example, responds directly to function and dysfunction. Lymph glands are scattered throughout the body, including between muscle fibers. The muscle is literally helping to pump the gland to effectuate lymphatic flow. Hence, inactive muscles impact on lymphatic function.**

The Ups and Downs of Shoulder Function

The key to defeating shoulder pain—and avoiding it altogether—is rediscovering function. I say "rediscovering" because functions are never totally lost. They are misplaced, sometimes for half a lifetime or more, but they can be found again, although it may take hard searching. Recently a client, K.C., told me that he probably hadn't been down on the floor in at least thirty years. As a result of his shoulder pain and other conditions, he could barely walk or hold himself upright. For his first few visits to the clinic, all we had him do was get on the floor and get up again. It wasn't easy for him, but after the first hour he was stronger and told me that he felt exhilarated. The amazing thing about these basic—lost—functions is that without them we are cheated of the joy we experienced as children, when climbing a tree or crawling on our hands and knees was pure fun. What K.C. was experiencing as exhilaration was a return to his youth. He was turning back the clock. The kinesthetic sense of how healthy motion feels, from the release of endorphins and the muscular interaction with the lymphatic system to increased respiration and circulation, kicked in. K.C. hadn't felt that way in years. And he wasn't running a marathon, he was moving a distance of about four feet.

Some muscles and joints have distinctive pain signatures, but the shoulders do not. Constant or intermittent, sharp or numb, tingling, burning, or throbbing—the characteristics are varied. Frequently stiffness takes the place of pain. At least twice a week a new client comes into the clinic with an encapsulated or "frozen" shoulder that doesn't hurt yet refuses to budge beyond a certain point. It doesn't matter whether there's stiffness or pain, almost every shoulder problem, with the exception of *serious* accidents resulting from high impact, is caused by the shoulder being out of proper position. Why is it out of position? The classic reason: Muscles have moved it there.

Therefore, before you seek treatment for shoulder pain, it is necessary to get a rough idea of what the shoulder joint is doing in relation to the *other* load-bearing joints. Most people don't realize it, but the shoulders are indeed load-bearing joints. They participate with the hips, knees, and ankles in supporting the full weight of the body. A shoulder, for exam-

> ### WAKE-UP CALL
>
> **Waking up in the middle of the night with tingling or numbness in your arms is often a symptom of shoulder misalignment. The structure is impeding the blood circulation. There can be more serious causes, but if the feeling returns quickly when you change position or move the limb, it stands to reason that musculoskeletal factors are involved.**

ple, will move forward to counterbalance an unstable hip that has slipped to the rear; its mate might move that way, too, or go in the opposite direction, or stay put. If we ignore that context and treat the shoulder in isolation, the problems will persist.

The first thing to do, then, is to get into the Static Back position (see chapter 5, figure 5–5, page 70) for a few minutes. Don't stay down long enough for gravity to flatten the back; in this case, we want to see what the muscles are doing with the bones. Determine if you have an arch in your lower back. Can you slip your hand under it? Next, assess the shoulders: Are they rounded up and off the floor, with the weight resting on the back of the head and the shoulder blades? If they are, do the following E-cises.

Total time: This menu can take a while because of the Progressive Supine Groin stretch. For severe pain, you may want to do this stretch for forty-five minutes to an hour. For slight pain, fifteen to twenty minutes will do.

Times a day: Once in the morning.

Duration: Do exercises daily until pain abates for twenty-four hours. Once the pain is gone, continue with the menu for one week before switching to the overall conditioning program in chapter 13. For nonpain symptoms such as bad posture, use this E-cise menu for three weeks, and then switch.

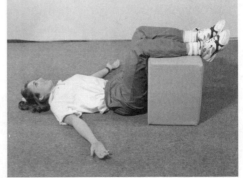

• 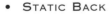 STATIC BACK

Follow the instructions for Static Back in chapter 5 (figure 5–5, page 70). Hold for at least twenty minutes as gravity flattens the back and hips.

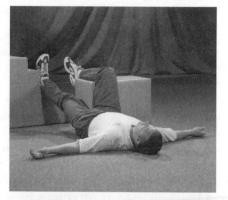

• PROGRESSIVE SUPINE
  GROIN

The instructions for
Progressive Supine Groin are
found in chapter 6 (figures
6–12 a and b, page 96). Don't
cheat; do it on both sides! This
E-cise encourages the powerful
groin muscles to release the
hip. Notice how the two
shoulders react differently to
this E-cise.

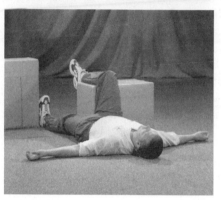

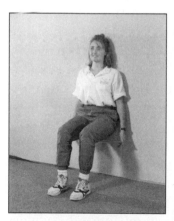

• AIR BENCH

Follow the instructions for Air Bench
in chapter 4 (figure 4–8, page 57). Keep
your shoulders back against the wall.
Press your hips, right and left, evenly
into the wall. Breathe. Hold for two minutes, building to three.
This E-cise allows vertical loading to take place while major
posture joint alignment is occurring.

TESTING THE SHOULDER'S BIFUNCTIONAL JOINT

Try it yourself: Remain seated, round your shoulders forward and down, tighten the muscles to hold them there, and raise your arms overhead. Can't get them up very far, eh? Put them out to the side and try again. Still tough. Notice, though, that the elbows don't seem to be affected—they are, but it's not obvious now. Thus, to get arm mobility and articulation, we shift functions from the shoulders to the elbows. At this stage, the rotator cuff works overtime and dysfunctionally—and painfully!—as it attempts to synchronize the rotation of the humerus and the scapula.

These E-cises should provide immediate pain relief unless you have a tear in the rotator cuff. The rotator cuff allows the shoulder to rotate via the ball-and-socket joint that holds the head of the arm's humerus bone. When you forcefully move your arms out of the range-of-motion box that we discussed earlier in this chapter, the musculature can be damaged if the shoulder rounds far enough forward to restrict rotational function. Splitting firewood with an ax, serving a tennis ball, and casting with a surf-fishing rod are just a few examples of rotational demands that the shoulder is designed to handle with ease—but that it cannot handle if it's stuck in the for-ward hinged position. The shoulder both hinges and rotates, but by living inside the box, the hinge becomes the predominant function, since, to meet most rotational demands, we end up using our elbows by flexing and extending the forearms.

The three E-cises that start on page 148 will suppress much of the active rotator cuff pain by removing the obstruction, but a torn rotator cuff means there's been tissue damage. In that case the heal-ing process will take more time, and until the damaged tissue mends, discomfort will linger in the area of one or both shoulder blades. Nevertheless, there's no way the rotator cuff will ever prop-erly recover until the restriction is eliminated. Surgical remedies that don't take this principle into account will fail. The E-cise menu realigns the shoulder structure and reactivates muscular function. Continue with the menu until the pain goes; then, switch to the conditioning routine in chapter 13 to maintain the progress you've made.

The next set of E-cises is for those who, when they do Static Back, find that their back is flat on the floor without an arch and that their shoulders are rounded up and off the floor. These conditions mean that we have to work on taking the flexion out of your back and hips in order to access your shoulder functions.

> **Total time: This menu can take a while because of the Supine Groin Stretch on Towels. For severe pain, you may want to do this stretch for forty-five minutes to an hour. For slight pain, fifteen to twenty minutes will do.**
> **Times a day: Once in the morning.**
> **Duration: Do exercises daily until pain abates for twenty-four hours. Once the pain is gone, continue with the menu for one week before switching to the overall conditioning program in chapter 13. For nonpain symptoms such as bad posture, use this E-cise menu for three weeks, and then switch.**

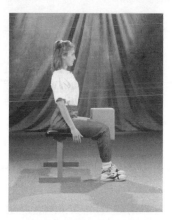

• SITTING KNEE PILLOW SQUEEZES

Follow the instructions for this E-cise in chapter 6 (figure 6–10, page 94). Keep your feet straight, and don't let your head and shoulders come forward. Do three sets of twenty. This E-cise gives the abductor/adductors something to do besides rotate the hip.

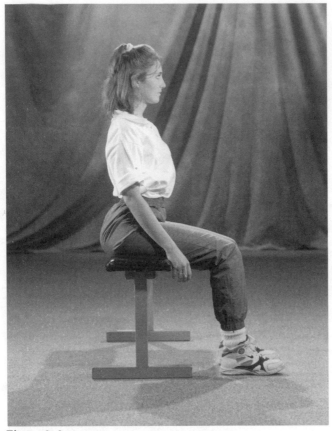

Figure 9–3

- SITTING SCAPULAR CONTRACTIONS
  (Figure 9–3)

Sit on the edge of a bench or chair with your hips in extension—
that is, rolled forward with your back arched and your head and
shoulders back. Slowly and evenly squeeze the shoulder blades
together, then release. Do three sets of twenty.

Frozen shoulder blades interfere with hip flexion-extension,
and this E-cise addresses the problem.

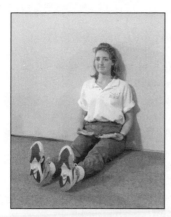

• SITTING FLOOR

Follow the instructions for Sitting Floor in chapter 6 (figure 6–11, page 95). Concentrate on making sure that your body is bilateral; don't work one side harder than the other. Hold the position for five minutes.

This E-cise forces a simple function to take place in a vertical state with the knees and ankles semiunloaded.

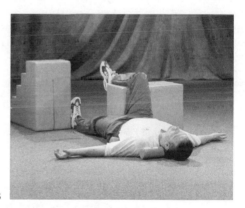

• SUPINE GROIN STRETCH ON TOWELS

Follow the instructions for this E-cise in chapter 6 (figure 6–8, page 92). The towels should keep your hips level from side to side. If we don't tame the groin muscles, they will continue to rotate the hips and with them the trunk. Hold for ten to fifteen minutes for each leg.

Hips: Elephant's Ears and Reclining Lounge Chairs

The pelvis has two crescent-shaped hipbones, one on the right side and the other on the left. Both of them attach to the sacrum, which is roughly triangular and forms a base for the spine to rest on. Together the bones of this pelvic structure, without flesh, look like the head of an elephant, viewed from the front. The two hips are the ears, while the sacrum has the outline of the animal's forehead, face, and trunk. The hips, like the elephant's ears, can move independently of each other; the right one swings forward while the left one remains in place or goes to the rear. In addition, the top of the hips can shift up or down independently, since there is a joint at the sacrum that allows for a certain amount of play. Moreover, the sacrum itself tips right and left, forward and back, which changes the positions of the hips (the way the elephant would waggle its head). Finally, the hips function like a pair of reclining lounge chairs. The lower ends swing out and up, the way footrests move, as the headrests tip back. Both go the other way as well, and they do so without regard to what position their partner is in. One can be forward and the other back, or both forward at the same time, or both back. All of this may seem confusing, but it makes perfect sense in terms of the body's design. The hip must assume many positions to function under many different demands. Problems arise when the hips stop moving freely from place to place and get stuck up or down, forward or back.

The final set of E-cises is for those whose chronic shoulder pain is caused by an elevated hip, an increasingly common condition in which one hip is repositioned higher than the other.

You can spot variations in your hip elevation by measuring the legs of a pair of trousers that have recently been altered for length. If one of them is longer than the other, the tailor has made an adjustment for the variation in hip position. Women often find, when they glance at a full-length mirror, that the bottom hems of their skirts are uneven; if it happens frequently to you, that's another indication that one hip is higher than the other. If your clothing doesn't tell you, maybe the bare facts will. Disrobe, stand before the mirror, place a thumb on each hipbone, and take a long, hard look. Still in doubt? You could have someone measure from each hipbone to the floor.

An elevated hip and chronic shoulder pain are basically pure cause and effect. Once the hip jams into an up or down position, the shoulder has to react. It moves up or down (or forward or back). Without stability in the load-bearing hip joint, the shoulder becomes unstable.

Whether it's the right or left hip that's elevated, these E-cises are appropriate.

> **Total time: This menu can take a while because of the Supine Groin Stretch on Towels. For severe pain, you may want to do this stretch for forty-five minutes to an hour. For slight pain, fifteen to twenty minutes will do.**
>
> **Times a day: Once in the morning.**
>
> **Duration: Do exercises daily until pain abates for twenty-four hours. Once the pain is gone, continue with the menu for one week before switching to the overall conditioning program in chapter 13. For nonpain symptoms such as bad posture, use this E-cise menu for three weeks, and then switch.**

• STANDING GLUTEAL CONTRACTIONS

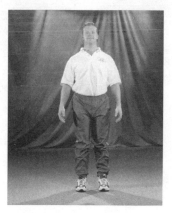 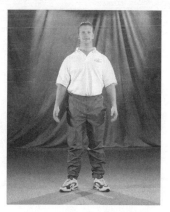

See the instructions for this E-cise in chapter 6 (figure 6–5, page 89). Be sure to use the buttocks muscles and not the thighs or abdominals. Do three sets of fifteen with your feet parallel and three sets of fifteen with your feet everted (out).

This E-cise reenegages the gluteal muscles.

- PRONE ANKLE SQUEEZES
  (Figure 9–4)

Lying on your stomach, rest your chin on your hands, and bend your knees to ninety degrees. Keep your knees slightly wider than your hips, and squeeze a pillow between your ankles, triggering the buttocks muscles evenly. Do three sets of fifteen.

This E-cise works the posterior and anterior muscles in tandem.

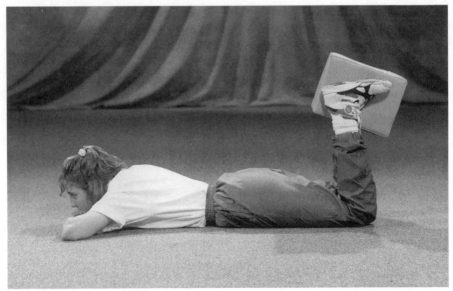

Figure 9–4

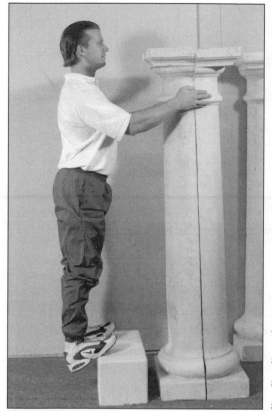

Figure 9–5

- GRAVITY DROP
  (Figure 9–5)

Wearing rubber-soled shoes for traction, stand on a step or stairway as though you were climbing upward. Your feet are parallel and shoulder-width apart. With one hand, hold on to the railing or another object for support, and edge backward until your heels are off the step and hanging in midair. Keep easing back so that more than half the foot is off the step. Make sure the feet remain parallel, pointing straight ahead, and that they are hip-width apart. Let the weight of your body press down into your heels to engage the posterior muscles of the leg. Don't bend the knees. Hold for three minutes.

This E-cise reengineers the linkage between the heel and all the joints straight up to the shoulders.

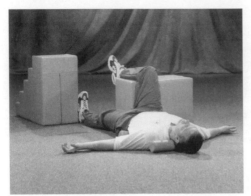

- SUPINE GROIN STRETCH
  ON TOWELS

Follow the instructions for this E-cise in chapter 6 (figure 6–8, page 92). Hold for ten to fifteen minutes for each leg. As the minutes tick by, you will feel the muscles in the front of your thigh taking over from the groin muscles.

In general, don't expect shoulder pain necessarily to be located on the same side of the body as the elevated hip; many times it is, but not always. The body has many ways to compensate for hip and shoulder instability. For example, the left shoulder and left hip may be elevated, and to compensate you swing the right shoulder forward and tighten the rotator cuff mechanism, which starts to hurt. In this case, the right hip would be the wrong place to look for elevation. Wherever it is, though, the E-cise treatment is the same.

Plain Geometry or Pain Geometry

Imagine the human trunk as being composed of two three-dimensional triangles, balanced tip to tip. One base forms the hips, and the other forms the shoulders (figure 9–6). This image gives you a sense of why joint interaction is so important. The powerful musculature that bridges and interconnects the triangles is constantly affecting the skeletal structure and, in turn, is being affected by it. Nothing happens in isolation. When we spend so much of our lives

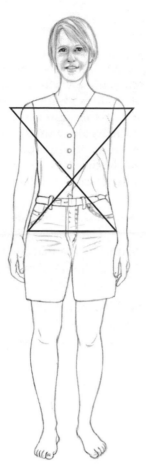

Figure 9–6
Triangles are a basic
musculoskeletal unit.

sitting down, the position of the hips inevitably takes on the shape
of a chair by moving to the rear and pulling the base of the lower triangle with it. The shoulders have no choice but to react, and it is
their reaction that has consequences.

A QUICK CHECK FOR SHOULDER RESTRICTIONS

Anytime you want to check on whether your shoulders are
aligned and bilateral, just try the following exercise. Stand up
with your feet pointed out like a duck, and roll your shoulders
forward. Then raise your right arm over your head and hold

it there for ten seconds. Lower the right arm, and do the
same for the left. If there was a detectable difference
between the two—if one arm felt heavier, stiffer, or the like—
you know you have a restriction in one shoulder that isn't in
the other. But even if they both felt the same, the shared
feeling was lousy, right? Now do it again, but this time
position the feet pigeon-toed and hold the shoulders back. It's
probably a lot easier this way on both sides. In the second
case, the hip is put into extension where it belongs; the lower
triangle's base comes forward.

A skeptic might say, "No matter how much my shoulder hurts,
I'm not going to stand around pigeon-toed all the time." You don't
have to. The stance merely duplicates mechanically what your mus-
cles are supposed to do to the hips naturally and automatically.
Those muscles need to be engaged and their functions restored.
When that happens, you're out of pain and out of the box.

10

ELBOWS, WRISTS, AND HANDS: THE MOVING FINGER . . .

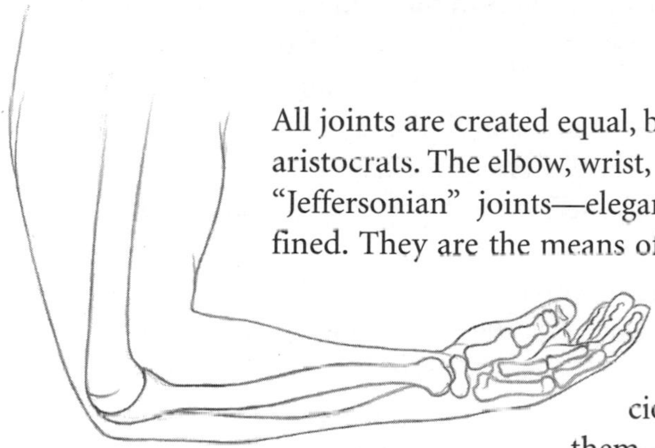

Figure 10–1

All joints are created equal, but some joints are true aristocrats. The elbow, wrist, and hand joints are the "Jeffersonian" joints—elegant, articulate, and refined. They are the means of writing sonnets, reattaching retinas, and flying space shuttles. There's nothing precious or fragile about them, though. The thumb and forefinger are where theory and experience converge. Capable of a light touch or a killing blow, praying or punching, these joints epitomize the ascent of man. When they hurt, we pay attention.

The Difference Between the Source and the Site of Pain

Cassie was paying close attention to her right wrist. She came to the clinic a few years ago because her wrist was in such a bad way. Stiff and painful, it had forced her to take an extended medical leave from her job as a social worker.

Cassie was a full hour into her first visit before she casually mentioned that her low back was also in extreme pain. Her priority was the wrist, however; everything else, she said, was of secondary importance. Like shoulder pain, pain in the elbow, wrist, or hands can be particularly disturbing. Beyond the discomfort, it also raises the prospects of job loss, a drastic change in lifestyle, and helplessness. She wanted to go back to work as soon as possible. As far as she was concerned, back pain wasn't going to interfere with that goal. She could either put up with it or do something about it later.

What Cassie didn't realize at first was that her wrist and low back pain were two different symptoms of the same problem: She had lost her vertical load-bearing capacity. Typically, she made the assumption that the site of the pain was also the source of the pain; I gave her a quick demonstration to convince her otherwise.

"Stand here with your toes pointed in," I requested. She moved her feet a little. "Come on, more than that. Really torque those knees and point them in." Her shoulders slumped, and she leaned forward at the waist. "The feet are perfect, but get the head and shoulders back—that's it."

"I feel like I'm going to topple to the right," she said.

"Don't worry, you won't. But the reason you feel that way is because most of your weight is being carried on the left side of your body, and this stance is redistributing it bilaterally. The right side isn't used to doing its fair share of the work." She nodded tentatively, still getting accustomed to the awkward position.

"How's your back feel?" I asked.

"Okay, I guess."

"Does it hurt?"

"Not right now."

"Does it usually hurt when you're standing?"

Cassie hesitated a moment. "Constantly."

"But it's not now?"

"No."

I gave her time to think about it. "How's the wrist?"

She raised her arm and took a look. The hand was held flat, palm down and fingers straight. "The same," she said.

"Try bending it." Cassie slowly clenched her fingers into a fist and opened them. Then she let her open hand droop down at the wrist and slowly—very slowly—flexed it upward. The hand stayed palm-out for about thirty seconds, then she quickly waggled it up and down, side to side, without saying a word.

"Well?" I asked finally.

"Wow!"

Cassie's problem wasn't in her wrist, elbow, or shoulder. Wrist braces and ergonomic keyboards weren't going to be of any help to her. Cassie's hip was causing her wrist pain. When I put her in the awkward stance, her statement that she felt like she was about to topple over to the right was an important piece of information. Lack of balance is always a message. In this instance it told me that her right hip was unstable; the turned-out right foot confirmed it and established that the

> **STRUCTURAL STRENGTH AND RESILIENCE**
>
> **Most chronic wrist pain is easily treated by returning the shoulder to alignment with the hip, knee, and ankle. Unless there is a bone fracture or traumatic joint dislocation, there is rarely structural damage.**

hip was tipped to the rear into flexion. To adjust the center of gravity and to walk in a straight line, Cassie unconsciously rotated her right shoulder forward and in. Without the underpinning from the load-bearing joints below, her shoulder sagged and compromised the ball-and-socket function.

The biomechanics are straightforward. As I pointed out in the last chapter, the shoulder is designed to both hinge and rotate. When its rotational capability is restricted, the elbow is recruited to handle the assignment. To get an idea of what's going on, extend your right arm in front of you, shoulder height, with the palm down. While keeping the arm straight, rotate it so that the palm is up. If you haven't lost shoulder function totally, the whole arm will move, and there will be detectable motion and muscular activity in the shoulder area as it participates in the rotation. With your other hand, gently squeeze up and down the length of the right arm, from the wrist to the shoulder, while doing this rotation. You'll feel many of the musculoskeletal mechanisms at work. Notice that the elbow itself rolls under in a semicircle. Now bend the elbow to ninety degrees,

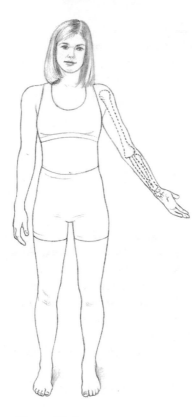

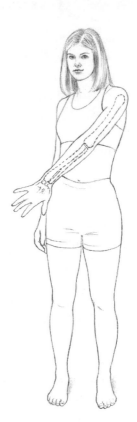

Figure 10–2
The ulna and radius as they
cross and as they lie parallel.

Figure 10–3
The palm in pronation.

tuck it into your side, and rotate the palm down and back up the same way. The shoulder is out of it, as are most of the muscles of the upper arm. The stationary elbow is working overtime by cranking hard on the ulna and the radius, the two bones of the forearm that are designed to go from lying parallel to each other to crossing one atop the other (figures 10–2 and 10–3).

Try this as well: Hold your hand out palm-down, and cross the middle finger over the top of the index finger. This movement roughly matches the movement of the radius in relation to the ulna as the forearm and wrist rotate. That forceful biomechanical *pas de deux* is repeated every time the hand and wrist move through their basic rotational range of motion. In addition, as it narrows toward the wrist, the musculoskeletal components of the forearm are compacted together anyway. With the extra rotation generated by the elbow, the bones, muscles, tendons, ligaments, and nerves don't have enough room to do their things without getting in each other's way. Rotation still occurs, but with increased friction. And friction does funny things. Rub two sticks together occasionally, and nothing happens; rub them together constantly, and there's a fire. When I asked Cassie about her elbow, she said there often was a burning sensation.

The Buck Stops Here—and There

The elbow, like the knee, is a synchronizing mechanism. As the knee works with the hip and ankle, the elbow coordinates and mediates the movement of the shoulder and the wrist. Like the knee, too, the elbow is a reduction gear. It translates the powerful movement of the shoulder into a form that the wrist and hand can use for controlled precision work. But if the shoulder is disconnected because

UNDERSTANDING WRIST AND ELBOW LINKAGE

To see and feel elbow misalignment in action, resume the position with the elbow bent at ninety degrees, tucked into your side, and with the palm up. Rotate the forearm palmdown, but make sure the elbow stays in place. Notice the tension on the inside of your wrist; the thumb doesn't want to come all the way over. Bring the thumb back until it is pointing straight up; if you try to stiffen the wrist, there isn't much strength and stability. The elbow is, in effect, telling the wrist that it's going to have to deal with the added rotational friction—that explains the tension on the inside of the wrist. As well, the inability to really lock the wrist hard comes from the elbow being deprived of the shoulder function required to roll it inward and upward, where it can stabilize and utilize the whole arm, upper torso, and back for the job.

of misalignment, the elbow must either make up for the lost shoulder power or pass the problem on down to the wrist. It does both.

The upper limbs draw their dynamic power from the musculoskeletal structure of the torso. The complexity of the muscular harmonization makes the interplay of a symphony orchestra seem simple. But most of us only use half our arms—the forearms. That means we've opened a biomechanical gap of about twelve inches between the elbow and the rest of the body. Blood flows and neural signals are transmitted through this zone (although those functions are compromised, too), but the full panoply of muscular and biomechanical activity is drastically reduced. Under the circumstances, wrist and elbow pain is inevitable.

A Transfer of Power

When it comes to range of motion, as I emphasized in the chapter on shoulder pain, most of us are locked into a three-by-four-foot box. Like the old-fashioned stocks that were used to punish petty criminals in the seventeenth and early eighteenth centuries, we've inserted our hands, wrists, arms, and shoulders into this box and confined them there for life. Notice how closely your elbows remain to the sides of your torso. Of the dozens of individual motions you perform in a given fifteen- or twenty-minute period, the elbows will only occasionally rise to anywhere near the level of the shoulders. We've contrived to put our work and play right in the middle of the box, from keyboards and steering wheels to computer games, TV remote-control devices, and mountain bikes. By doing so, we have turned the elbow, wrist, and hand into the drudges of the upper half of the body. When the musculoskeletal design is working properly, just bending forward at the waist causes the torso's flexion-extension capability to nearly double the reach of our arms. But when it isn't working properly—and wrist and elbow pain tell us when it is not—that faculty is transferred to the elbows, wrists, and hands, along with lateral and rotational movement of the trunk.

The hips and torso remain in place while the elbow shifts position to execute an infinite number of routine moves. Meanwhile,

ISOLATING THE WRISTS AND ELBOWS LEADS TO CHRONIC PAIN

Stop a moment to focus on the consequences to the elbows, wrists, and hands of the chain of dysfunction that runs from the hips to the shoulders. Nearly all of the trunk's major muscles and biomechanical structures are compromised. Their work is being shifted to the elbows, wrists, and hands. Imagine reaching out to lift a heavy dictionary from a shelf in front of you that's chest-high and three feet away. If your hips are already in forward flexion, the arm will be used to cover the distance instead of bending at the waist to shorten the distance between you and the bookcase. Since your shoulder is rounded forward it cannot support the weight of the volume, so it relies on the elbow and wrist. This sequence is repeated hundreds of times a day. Chronic pain is inevitable.

shoulders that are designed to help push, pull, stretch, and lift are rounded forward and inert. The job of moving any weight is delegated to the elbows and wrists. That would be no problem in a fully functional body. It's one of the reasons why we have powerful biceps and triceps muscles (as well as the other flexor-extensor muscles of the arms). But in a body that's "boxed in" and has shoulder dysfunction and pain, the arm muscles' capacity to participate in a full range of motion—on the order of hoisting and lowering the forearm through an arc of 165 degrees—is reduced to a third to a half of what it should be. Lifting a coffee cup or glass to the lips and setting it down again become major challenges.

It's not just lifting, pushing, and pulling that are curtailed. Pronation and supination of the forearms need shoulder involvement. Without the shoulder, most of the function takes place in the elbow and wrist. The positions that our hands are in determine the kind of work we do and, ultimately, who we are. For example, take a classic scene from a drawing-room comedy or a *Masterpiece Theater* costume drama: A country bumpkin is invited to a posh drawing room for tea. He brings the delicate bone china cup to his lips by lifting his elbow until it is as high as his ear. Meanwhile, the hostess flutters her eyelashes in disapproval, and the host sneers. The elegant couple raise their own cups with their elbows demurely tucked in and down. The Regency redneck has shoulder function, while his lordship and her ladyship do not. He accomplishes pronation of the hand with his shoulder, elbow, and wrist; they are mostly using their wrists.

> ## PRONATION AND SUPINATION
>
> The same terms are used for important functions in both the foot/ankle and the forearm. They derive from *prone* and *supine*. If you lie on your stomach, you are prone; roll over on your back, and you are supine. When the forearm pronates, the palm of the hand faces down (if the elbow is at a ninety-degree angle), or it faces toward the rear (when the arms are at the sides).

Do we unconsciously associate dysfunctional and functional physical characteristics with certain social groups? Indeed we do, and ironically it is many of the dysfunctions that are regarded as cool and stylish. Every spring- and fall-fashion season, I'm again struck by the "look" that designers create using models who grow ever more stoop-shouldered, whose heads hang, and whose torsos tip forward. They slouch down the runways in Paris, New York, and London with their feet everted and their hips rolled back into flexion.

The next time you're watching a fashion show, notice that as the models approach, the backs of their hands are pointed straight ahead. It is evidence of shoulder disengagement. Without proper design movement in the shoulder blades and the humerus bones of the upper arms, their forearms and wrists rotate inward. The pronator muscles of the forearms are put into flexion; as a result, they are engaged in the crossing motion with the radius and ulna that I mentioned earlier. It means that the wrist, forearm, and elbow operate in maximally constricted and congested conditions. The musculoskeletal structure never returns to a neutral position. Extra friction is constant. Combustion—pain—is sure to follow.

The Perils and Pain of Doctor Shopping

The body tries to extinguish the fire in a variety of ways. One way is to secrete fluids that limit the friction by acting as cushions and braking mechanisms. This secretion happens in the elbow's synovial joint. Pouches or cysts of snyovial fluid will form behind the elbow, making it difficult to bend or rotate the joint. Some people get their elbows "drained" as frequently as they change the oil in the family car—a little more painfully, though.

Likewise, the bursal sacs, which are strategically placed at friction points (that is, where tendons contact bones), fill up and restrict movement. The sheathing on the tendons themselves can become raw and inflamed, and sometimes the tendon even "slips." This condition is called epicondylitis, but the tendon is not really slipping; rather, compensating muscles are repositioning the bones in relation to the tendon. The surgical remedy is to find another route for the tendon, one that offers less friction. But this approach only increases the elbow dysfunction, because the joint was designed to have the tendon in its original location.

The fire department's primary weapon is to shut down the joint by making it too painful to move. As the elbow and wrist become stiff, restricted, and painful, movement is slowly diminished. We all instinctively know that this is a last resort remedy, and in the short run, the friction abates. The elbow and wrist, however, are so central to our modern lives that losing full use of them is a major crisis. As a result, the usual pattern over the long run is a period of relative elbow or wrist inactivity in order to quell pain symptoms, followed by a resumption of the demand that caused the friction in the first place. Gradually the relief gained during the periods of inactivity dwindles to the vanishing point, while the pain becomes constant.

Our usual compulsion is to "play through the pain." The best example of that attitude is a handball champion who came to me several years ago, as his last resort, for help with a sore elbow. For years, in order to continue playing, he had been receiving regular cortisone shots. Any competent physician will tell you that the words *regular* and *cortisone* should not appear in the same sentence. Cortisone can be potent as a pain-killer, but repeated doses have serious side effects. This man, Gil, apparently had shopped around for doctors who would agree to give him the shots without asking too many questions. When they refused to provide second and third helpings, he would go elsewhere. Eventually, the excess cortisone caught up to him. When I first saw Gil, he was desperate to play in a major tournament despite agonizing pain. He admitted he had had many cortisone shots and that he was turning to me because no doctor would agree to administer another one.

"Why not?" I asked.

"Feel my elbow."

I took his right elbow and gently squeezed it. As I did so, my thumb slid up and into the joint, pushing the skin before it as though I were slipping into a glove. The elbow is an impressive triple joint, packed with cartilage, ligaments, bone condyles, and tendons. But my thumb went into Gil's elbow past the knuckle. Gil's elbow joint mechanism, thanks to the cortisone, had collapsed. The pain-killer had allowed him to keep playing year after year while the bone and other tissue were reduced to mush. Sadly, there was nothing I could do for Gil. It is very difficult to treat elbow pain when there is no elbow joint left. He had opted to kill the pain, to override its message, and ended up killing his elbow.

HOT SPOTS

Friction in or near joints will produce hot spots. You can feel them with the palm of your hand; sometimes there's a visible blotch of red, too. These may not hurt, but they are symptoms of dysfunction that shouldn't be ignored. The E-cises for the nearest major joint will help.

Elbow Pain Treatment

Few of us are that fanatical about playing through the pain or foolish enough to abuse cortisone; it's probably safe to assume that your elbow is still alive. These five E-cises are designed to restore the linkage between the elbow, shoulder, torso, and hip. As with the E-cises in each chapter, do them all in the order presented.

Total time: This menu can take a while because of the Supine Groin Stretch. For severe pain, you may want to do this stretch for forty-five minutes to an hour. For slight pain, fifteen to twenty minutes will do.

Times a day: Once in the morning.

Duration: Do exercises daily until pain abates for twenty-four hours. Once the pain is gone, continue with the menu for one week before switching to the overall conditioning program in chapter 13.

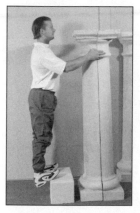

• GRAVITY DROP

Follow the instructions for Gravity Drop in chapter 9 (figure 9–5, page 157). Make sure your feet are parallel and pointing straight ahead; they may try to evert. Concentrate on equalizing your weight on both sides, and press into the heels. Hold for three minutes. Imagine that your heels and head are up against an invisible wall. This pulls your torso, shoulders, and head back into alignment with the hips.

• STATIC EXTENSION

Follow the instructions for Static Extension in chapter 4 (figure 4–7, page 56). Work on allowing the shoulder blades to come together. Also, it's important to let your head hang down; make sure the neck and upper back muscles are relaxed. Hold for one minute, building to two minutes.

Static Extension takes the C out of your spine and reminds the shoulder joint that it's supposed to hinge forward *and* back.

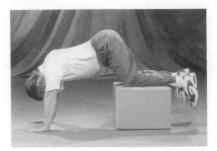

* CIRCUMDUCTION
  (Figure 10–4)

You'll need a low bench that will allow you to stand beside it with one leg straight and the other bent at ninety degrees while resting on the surface of the bench. Bend at the waist, placing the hand that is opposite the straight leg palm-down on the bench for support. Position a five-pound weight under the free hand, where

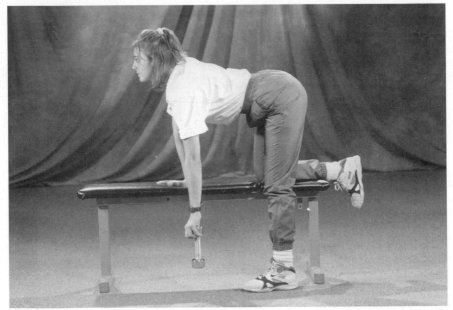

Figure 10–4

you can reach down and pick it up. The weight should be in a vertical position so that you can grasp its head. Hold the weight lightly—don't clench your hand or throw your arm muscles into a hard contraction—as you gently swing the fully extended arm in a small circle. Let the momentum carry the arm through the circle. Your arm isn't "windmilling" up and over the head and around; it's inscribing small, easy circles on the floor. Circle twenty times clockwise, and twenty times counterclockwise, then repeat on the other side. Do two sets of thirty for each arm.

Circumduction restores the ball-and-socket function to a shoulder joint that has frozen into the forward hinged position.

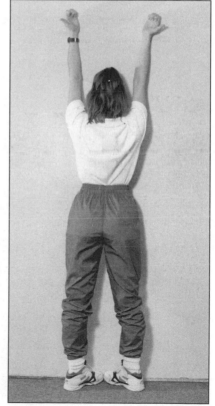

- WALL CLOCK
  (Figure 10–5 a, b, and c)

This is a three-position E-cise. You should feel it in the shoulder's AC process (the joint mechanism where the humerus meets the clavicle and scapula) and the shoulder blades. If position three aggravates your elbow pain, drop it from the sequence initially. Try it again after a day or two of doing positions one and two; when it no longer brings on pain, add it to the others.

Figure 10–5a

Position one (figure 10–5a): Face the wall, and place your feet in a pigeon-toed position up against the wall. Place your arms over your head in the twelve o'clock position, and hold for one minute. Your elbows are straight, while your shoulders are rotated away from the wall, with the thumbs pointing away from the wall. Hold for one minute.

Position two (figure 10–5b): Remain in the same pigeon-toed stance. Place your arms over your head in the ten-of-two position. Your elbows are straight, while your shoulders are rotated away from the wall, with the thumbs pointing away from the wall. Hold for one minute.

Position three (figure 10–5c): Remain in the same stance. Place your arms over your head in the quarter-to-three position. Your elbows are straight, while your shoulders are rotated away from

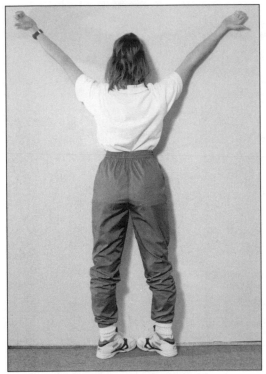

the wall, with the thumbs pointing away from the wall. Hold for one minute.

Wall Clock goes after the scapula. The shoulder blades are supposed to move—up and down, back and forth, and in clockwise and counterclockwise rotation. When they don't, much of the dynamic interaction with the torso is lost, and half of the shoulder's biomechanical capacity is unavailable.

Figure 10–5b

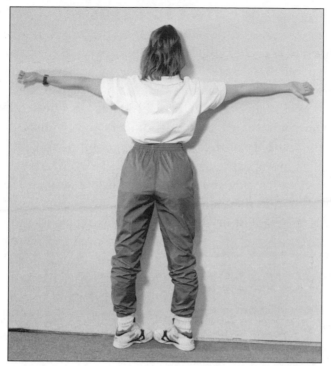

Figure 10–5c

• SUPINE GROIN STRETCH

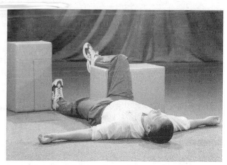

The instructions for Supine Groin Stretch are also in chapter 5 (figure 5–7, page 72). The problem here is underdoing it. Give the E-cise plenty of time to work. Hold for at least ten minutes per side. The groin muscles are powerful, and it takes time to persuade them to let go.

Wrists and Hands

I've deliberately pushed the subject of carpal tunnel syndrome (CTS) deep into this chapter to force readers who have its symptoms to confront what's really causing their pain. CTS is not caused by what we do with our elbows, wrists, or hands—it's caused by what we *don't* do. By not engaging the shoulders and by disrupting the load-bearing capacity of the body, our upper limbs and extremities are fighting a losing battle against pain. They do not have access to the nuanced muscle power and biomechanical interaction required to stay healthy. And there's no substitute for those functions. None. That's why the ergonomic redesign of the workplace—and of garden tools, toys, and mattresses—borders on fraud. Installing a wrist brace on a keyboard or raising the surface of a workbench only shifts the excess friction to another location in the worker's elbow, wrist, or hand. Before long, the friction will reignite the "fire." Like Gil's cortisone shots, workers are able to keep earning paychecks thanks to ergonomic inventiveness, but their musculoskeletal structures continue to deteriorate under the stress of the dysfunctions they bring to the job. Ergonomic palliatives are just as deadly as overdosing on painkillers.

> ### EAT, DRINK—AND MOVE
>
> **Just as we spend about an hour a day eating or eight hours sleeping, it is now necessary to take time out of the day to refuel our bodies with enough motion to maintain basic musculoskeletal functions.**

Aside from flagrantly unsafe or inhuman practices and severe accidents, workplace tasks are being unfairly blamed for causing injuries that are really symptoms of musculoskeletal dysfunction. These conditions can be readily corrected by any person willing to give his or her body a little *motional* nourishment.

The environment won't do it for us—not because of heartless employers, but because the amazing and abundant lives we have built for ourselves as twenty-first-century men and women no longer automatically provide enough motion to keep us healthy.

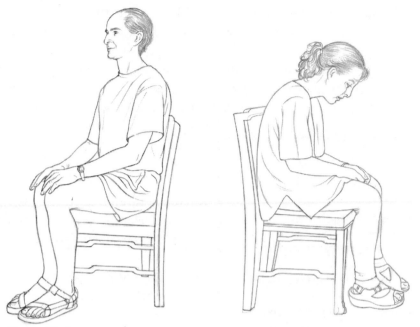

Figure 10–6

Two models, one functional, the other with symptoms of carpal tunnel syndrome.

Taking responsibility for motion is not about building big muscles or undergoing brutal workouts. Look at figure 10–6 to see what carpal tunnel pain is really about. The model on the left is functional: He's bilateral, the weight is distributed equally left to right, the load-bearing joints are in vertical alignment, and the horizontal lines run parallel through those joints. For most of us, this functional condition doesn't happen naturally anymore, and he's had to work at it himself. The model on the right offers a far different configuration. A friend of mine who saw this book as it was being written thought the comparison was jarring. She said, "Nobody looks that bad." We went for a walk around the office park where the clinic is located, and within fifteen minutes she had seen a couple dozen people who looked "that bad." I could have stopped any of them at random to answer a few questions and heard, "Yes, my wrist has been stiff lately," or "I get pains in my forearms." In these drawings, and in real life, the head, shoulder, and arm position explain what's happening with carpal tunnel syndrome.

Start with the rounded spine. Draw up close to your desk or a tabletop. Let your shoulders and back slump, and put your arms palm-down on the surface, elbows bent at ninety degrees and tucked in close to your torso. The wrists should be flat on the table. Slowly arch your spine and pull your head back (leave the shoulders where they are). Notice how your forearms elevate and lift your wrists off the table. That is, the position of your back is affecting the position of your wrists. Arching the back alone decreases friction in the wrists and positions them to accomplish extension of the fingers smoothly rather than pushing the mechanism further into flexion (i.e., flattening the wrist).

TYPE WITH YOUR SHOULDERS

The more shoulder involvement in typing, the better. Assist the muscles of the hand, wrist, and forearm by engaging the upper back and shoulder muscles. Strike the keys forcefully—even though your touch-typing teacher wouldn't approve. And don't pull the backs of your hands up and toward the wrists as you type; that obstructs the tendons.

Now consider your shoulders. Slumped forward, they position the arms via the elbows into permanent pronation—only the wrists would rather not be in permanent pronation. They want to rotate outward to allow the hands to grasp (rather than claw). The pronation creates friction that is compounded by the countervailing supination. As the hand moves, a whipsawing action back and forth between the pronator and supinator muscles stresses the wrist. Put your hands on a computer keyboard, and you may notice that they want to roll outward instead of remaining flat over the keys. If your shoulders are engaged, they will assist in pronating the hand; disengaged, the elbow and wrist must perform that role, and the result is extra friction.

Try another experiment. Scoot up close to your desk, bend your arms at the elbows to ninety degrees, and place the palms and wrists flat on the surface; let your back and shoulders slump forward. Raise your hands off the table and flex them back while keeping the wrists in place, and do that four or five times. The muscular and mechanical work that produced this motion was probably being performed underneath the wrists, where there is so little room to maneuver that the tendons are being rubbed raw. If you arch the back and pull your shoulders square, the same action will shift to the upper end of your forearms, where it belongs.

One more experiment. While your arms are flat on the table, bring your head down close to the surface so that you can see the arch under your right wrist. If it's not there, bob your right shoulder up and down a little; a space will open underneath the wrist where the meaty part of the palm begins. Rolling your shoulder down and in toward the back of the hand will press this arch flat into the table. The same thing is happening when the shoulder is in the forward hinged position and the hand is typing or playing the piano. Modern keyboards, including pianos, have such a light touch that our arms and shoulders are not being asked to participate in striking the keys. Consequently, the downstroke of the finger is being executed almost entirely by the finger muscles. Those muscles have bellies located in the forearm that reduce the mass of the hand and keep it flexible. By obstructing the routes that tendons travel past the carpal bones of the hands to get to the fingers—and that's what's happening when the wrist arch flattens—we are scraping the tendons across bone with every twitch of the fingers.

The primary cause of carpal tunnel syndrome is the same as the cause of generic wrist and elbow pain. It's too bad we give fancy names to symptoms that are related to the site of the pain instead of the source. In order to get well and stay that way, we must learn to be skeptical of any chronic pain treatment that narrowly focuses on the joint or area that is hurting.

Is It Really Arthritis?

I have mentioned arthritis in other chapters, but it also needs to be addressed here since the condition can impact on the elbows, wrists, and hands. One thing that should be understood about arthritis is that once it establishes itself in a joint by causing inflammation and tissue deterioration, the effects are normally relatively constant. What I mean is that arthritis—whatever it is that causes pain, stiffness, and swelling—does not as a rule turn on and then off. It's just there all the time. Why then does arthritis pain, in fact, come and go? Because in many cases arthritis pain is really muscular pain. When I work with clients who have arthritis, I invariably find that the pain they believe to be arthritic in nature can be turned off by altering the config-uration of their musculoskeletal structure. I have them do fifteen or twenty minutes of specific E-cises (the ones included later in this chapter). As far as I'm concerned, while that's no cure for arthritis, it's a lot better than living with debilitating pain or the se-rious side effects of drugs and surgical treatments.

> ## THE DANGER OF WRIST BRACES
>
> **Like knee braces, wrist braces should be avoided. They can never fully immobilize the structure, only limit and change the nature of the movement. The new pattern is also driven by muscular dysfunction. Plus, in the case of the wrist, the radius and ulna move in a different relationship to the humerus at the elbow joint. This isn't solving the problem, it's shifting it to the elbow.**

A few years ago, during a break in a business meeting in New York, I noticed a young woman off to one side of the room. She was in obvious pain, although she was doing her best to hide it. "Your hands hurt, don't they?" I asked. She nodded, the fingers of both hands slowly clenching. "Have you seen a doctor?"

She smiled. "Try doctors with an *s*. Zillions of doctors. I've had arthritis since I was a little girl."

"The pain is worse in the knuckles, right?"

"Right. And they're killing me now."

"Want it to stop?" By that point several of the meeting partici-pants had gathered around, and she was embarrassed. All I got in re-ply was a nervous shrug. "Please give me your hand," I said. She held it out. I tugged gently on the index finger. "Hurt?" She nodded. I tugged on the next one. "Hurt?" Again she nodded, and she did so each time as I repeated the procedure with the rest of her fingers. I then asked her to stand pigeon-toed and to pull her shoulders back as she arched her back.

I continued holding her hand and pulled on the index finger. "Hurt?"

"No."

The next one. "Hurt?"

She hesitated. "No."

Again. "Hurt?"

"Nope."

When I finished, her eyes were teary, but not from pain. "What does that tell you about the pain in your hands?"

She looked down at them. "It's not caused by the arthritis."

And she was absolutely right. While the woman did have arthritis in her hands, most of the pain came from muscular compensation and dysfunction. Her hands and wrists were getting no help from her disengaged shoulders. She and millions of other people with arthritis unconsciously limit and manage the way their bodies move in response to the condition. Over time, the result is acute muscular pain that is far more treatable than the mystery illness we call arthritis. I believe that the use of drugs could be curtailed and physical abilities restored to many arthritis sufferers by a program centered on musculoskeletal dysfunctions.

By way of confirmation, in 1996 an eighteen-month clinical study funded by the National Institute on Aging found that a program of moderate exercise—one hour, three times a week—for people with osteoarthritis of the knee resulted in less pain, reduced disability, and improved physical performance. The results, as reported in the *American Journal of Medicine,* were described as "modest but consistent." I would argue that if correcting musculoskeletal dysfunctions had also been included in the program, the improvement would have been dramatic, just like what I see all the time in my clinic. Without that extra correction, the study's results were diluted by the least functional participants, whose knees operated in ways that produced pain and restriction that were mistakenly assumed to be symptoms of arthritis. The idea is to get the friction and stress out of the joint, to allow its proper biomechanical interaction to take place. The functional musculoskeletal system has an amazing capacity to "manage" joint articulation in spite of major obstacles. We shouldn't assume that arthritis is the exception to this rule.

Treatment for Wrist and Hand Pain

In the three E-cises for wrist and hand pain, we'll reestablish the kinetic chain linking the hand, wrist, elbow, and shoulder; release and reposition the hip; and bring the hips, shoulders, and head into alignment. This menu will help with carpal tunnel syndrome, arthritis, and other chronic wrist and hand pain symptoms discussed in this chapter.

> **Total time: This menu can take a while because of the Supine Groin Stretch on Towels. For severe pain, you may want to do this stretch for forty-five minutes to an hour. For slight pain, fifteen to twenty minutes will do.**
> **Times a day: Once in the morning.**
> **Duration: Do exercises daily until pain abates for twenty-four hours. Once the pain is gone, continue with the menu for one week before switching to the overall conditioning program in chapter 13.**

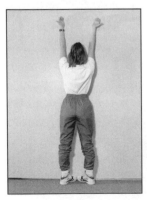

• WALL CLOCK

Follow the instructions for Wall Clock (figure 10–5 a, b, and c, page 173). Spend one minute in each position. By listening to what this E-cise is telling you, the link between all the load-bearing joints, from shoulder to ankle, will become obvious.

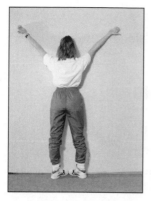

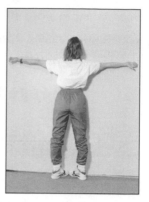

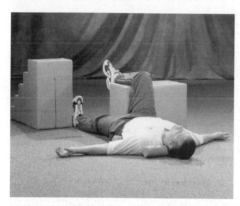

- ### Supine Groin Stretch on Towels

Follow the instructions for this E-cise in chapter 6 (figure 6–8, page 92). Hold for three minutes on each side. This E-cise seems time-consuming and passive, but it is extremely beneficial. By taming the powerful hip adductor and abductor muscles, it allows the hip to reposition.

- ### Air Bench

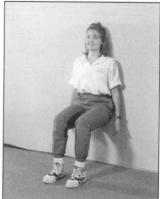

Follow the instructions for Air Bench in chapter 4 (figure 4–8, page 57). Hold for one minute, building to two minutes. As Air Bench becomes easier to do, you should congratulate yourself for making significant progress. It's strengthening your hip extensors, which had been outgunned by your flexor-rotational muscles. At the same time, your ankles, knees, and shoulders are being brought into line.

Responding to an Epidemic

Finally, a few words about a new class of conditions known as repetitive motion injuries (carpal tunnel syndrome is one of them), which have been officially described as "epidemic" in the workplace by the Labor Department. The joints of the human body were designed to move repetitively. There is no scientific evidence that our joints have a set, finite capacity for movement. The term *repetitive motion injury* implies that we hurt ourselves by moving a joint too many times in succession. But that's impossible because simple muscle fatigue sets in long before a healthy joint mechanism is damaged. What's actually happening with so-called repetitive motion injuries is that unstable joints, joints that have lost their kinetic connections, are moving too many times. Under those circumstances, any motion, let alone repetitive motion, is injurious. It's just a matter of how fast the musculoskeletal systems break down. An "accident" will happen—except we'll call it a repetitive motion injury. The remedy is to stabilize the joints, not to sedate or surgically reconfigure them. If you think you're developing pain symptoms of repetitive motion, the E-cises in this chapter for the specific joint (and the other chapters for the other joints) offer a major step toward stabilization.

It may well be that the hands, wrists, and elbows are the joints that will allow us to escape from the box. When they send a message, as they did to my client Cassie, any of us would pay attention. Among the many joints in the human body to which we rarely give a second thought, the hands, wrists, and elbows are truly up close and personal. Creatures who evolved from surviving on two feet to surviving with two hands that are extensions of experience, imagination, and will cannot allow hand function to be fatally compromised. This hope leads me back to the reason I refer to them as the "Jeffersonian" joints.

NECK AND HEAD:
ON THE LEVEL

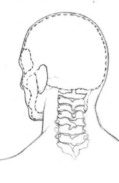

Figure 11–1

Years ago, in big-city department stores, the elevator operators would call out the specialties of each floor as the doors rumbled open like stiff curtains drawing back to reveal a new magic realm: "Household linens, notions, perfume, ladies' lingerie. . . ." As we arrive at the body's top floor, it seems appropriate to announce, "Neck pain and stiffness, dizziness, vertigo, headaches, TMJ—and more."

Not very inviting, is it? Instead of standing on a threshold looking out at a rich emporium, we are staring downward, straight into the infamous box, the same one I described in chapter 9. Only now, along with our hands, wrists, elbows, and shoulders, our neck and head are also being pulled toward confinement in the three-by-four-foot area directly in front of us that increasingly defines the modern range of motion. Despite their preeminent positions in the anatomical hierarchy, despite our own obsession with big brains and beautiful faces, the neck and the head are followers rather than leaders. They've gone along for the ride, from function to dysfunction; from pain free to painful; from heads up to hunkered down.

What's Happening to the Neck
and Head—and Why?

As the musculoskeletal system ascends past the thoracic back, its load-bearing capacity becomes more and more dependent on a stable foundation of muscles, joints, and bones. Above the shoulders, an intricate balancing act takes place without the direct assistance, by and large, of the major muscle groups and other structures of the hips and torso. This arrangement makes sense. Based on the assumption that the vertical integrity of the spine will counteract gravity, the neck's limited musculature is designed to handle a comparatively modest task: to move the head from front to back, and from side to side. Heavy lifting and lateral support do not figure all that much in the scheme of things. But our modern lives of minimal motion are encouraging the spine to move into forward flexion, distorting its S-curve into a C, and forcing the mechanisms of the neck to do hard labor in order to keep us from losing our heads. With the head tilted forward, gravity has us by the nose and is pulling. As a consequence, the cervical spine, the section between the shoulders and the base of the skull, may well be doing the most momentous work of any part of the musculoskeletal system, with the fewest resources.

The price? To quote the anatomical elevator operator, "Neck pain and stiffness, dizziness, vertigo, headaches, TMJ—and more." Nevertheless, neck and head position are consistently underrated, even ignored, as important causes of conditions ranging in severity from mildly irritating to immediately life-threatening. The time has come to stop merely looking at the head and to start really seeing it, reading it, and understanding what it is telling us.

In the clinic, my therapists and I often test ourselves by putting a new client's intake form off to one side without reading their reason for coming to us. "Have you taken a bad fall lately?" one of us might ask.

"As a matter of fact, just the other—"

Or we ask, "Do you have headaches?"

"Yes. Migraines every couple of weeks."

Our questions come from observing that the client's head and neck are out of position, losing the struggle with gravity.

Practical people who would never consider operating an appliance or power tool upside down or tipped at an angle, think nothing of asking their necks and heads to function at anywhere from five to forty-five degrees askew. The amazing thing about the human body is that it is capable of working under conditions that would quickly destroy man-made designs. We hardly think twice about stretching, straining, and assuming awkward positions to clean the attic, change the transmission fluid, or put up the Christmas lights. It's part of our ingrained behavior because we're programmed in a musculoskeletal sense—we have muscle memory—to respond to the ongoing demands of the environment. For millions of years, we've been able to successfully respond to these demands, ranging from the simple to the complex, from the customary to the contorted, because our basic musculoskeletal design was intact and functional. Today that essential requirement has been compromised; the neck and head position confirm the bad news.

> **NEUTRALITY**
>
> **All functional joints return to a neutral starting point. Dysfunctional joints stay engaged, either in flexion, extension, or a rotational mode. This loss of neutrality creates biomechanical conflict and pain.**

It's easy to crane your neck forward and down while making a precision adjustment of a valve. It's fully within the body's capability.

But to hold that position for weeks, months, and years at a time is another matter. To assume atypical postures and perform in them, the body recruits mechanisms that may not normally be involved in day-to-day movement. The more atypical the movement, the more the body must improvise; medical science has never catalogued all the possible combinations and probably never will. Suppose the valve is small and needs fine calibration. To steady your hand, your arm extends with the shoulder forward so that the scapula locks and helps stabilize the wrist. Meanwhile, the head comes forward to give the eyes a closer perception of the work; flexion in the thoracic back reduces the area of expansion for the diaphragm muscle under the lungs, and thus respiration becomes shallow, which serves to dampen extra vibration. This sequence gets the job done. If the body doesn't release the recruited mechanisms afterward and return to the neutral position, the musculoskeletal structure gets stuck in a specialized configuration. To go back to picking up heavy suitcases, reaching to the top shelf in the pantry for a can of peaches, or typing means using the wrong "tools." The neck and the head, tipped over as if to examine precision work, take a beating.

Overdoing precision work, or any type of work, is not the problem. Long before you ever had to set that valve, forward flexion of the spine and the other mechanisms of the trunk tipped your neck and head into that posture, where they remain, causing a long list of physical afflictions as you go about the imprecise business of working and playing. Due to the dysfunction, the body's unique ability to improvise is kicking in, not just for the specialty assignments but for the routine stuff.

In the motion sequence for adjusting the valve, the head is very much involved. That is a crucial point. The head weighs about ten pounds. That doesn't seem like much, but try this: Heft a ten-pound hand-weight or something similar straight over your head; hold it there with the arm fully extended. You'll find that the more vertical your arm, the easier it is to support the weight. Now, tip the weight slightly forward, and see how much more strain is created. As you bring it forward by degrees, the effort intensifies. This is exactly what's happening to the neck as it moves the head forward and down.

When Abbie came to the clinic, her neck and head were thrust so far forward that she had lost almost all her ability to turn them from side to side. In addition, it was impossible for her to look upward by tipping her head backward. It had happened gradually: Living in an affluent suburban environment, she was trapped in the box that we've discussed. Without noticing—and without needing to notice—she had slowly robbed herself of these important functions. What started out as a slight stiffness when she turned to look over her shoulder, then became a minor crick in the neck, which then froze in place as the years went by.

When my therapists started working with Abbie, they had her do the E-cise called Static Back (chapter 5, figure 5–5, page 70), using towels. Towels, rolled to the thickness of a fist, are sometimes used in this E-cise in case the lumbar and cervical curves need support. To our consternation, not even two of our thickest foam-rubber wedges were enough to support Abbie's head, since her neck and head were cranked forward a good four inches. We had to use another piece of foam-rubber equipment, this one built like a stepladder, so she could rest her head and neck on the first step. After about thirty minutes the E-cise released her neck, but her new position was so strange, she went into severe spasms. Her hip and back muscles had totally forgotten what they were supposed to do in that design position. The spasms were quickly brought under control. As unpleasant as they were, however, they served to explain to Abbie why she had needed rotator cuff surgery the year before and why her knees and back had been suffering from chronic pain. Today her pain is gone, and

> ## ERGONOMIC CHAIRS
>
> **These chairs are substituting their design for your muscles. They hold you in a position that forces the spine into a semblance of an S-curve, which is what your muscles are supposed to be doing but aren't. This does nothing to strengthen the muscles. When you stand up, the structures go right back into a dysfunctional position. Moreover, the chairs are so uncomfortable that people stop using them or figure out a way to defeat the design.**

when she visits the clinic for periodic checkups, she uses towels, not wedges or foam blocks cut like stepladders. Better yet, she can turn her head right and left, up and down.

The basic structure of the neck, otherwise known as the cervical spine, is more or less the same as that of the lumbar and thoracic spines. Vertebrae are stacked one atop the other, separated by disks, the tough, shock-absorbing pads of tissue. The spinal cord runs through a narrow central canal. But in the cervical spine this canal gets markedly smaller as it nears the base of the skull. It's smaller, that is, compared to the roomier passageway below, with its many apertures from which the central nervous system branches off profusely into the nooks and crannies of the torso and the lower extremities. Given the limited space, the cervical vertebrae are not able to flex and extend to the same degree as their lumbar and thoracic compatriots; they have neither the necessary mass nor the musculature.

Since it doesn't have much counterbalancing flexibility, the neck has little choice but to obey the hips. The forward flexion of the body, which starts primarily in the hips because we sit so much, reverses the cervical curve from convex to concave. This shift brings the head out of vertical alignment, where it was dynamically linked to and supported by the shoulders, hips, knees, and ankles. The spine goes from solid pedestal to flexible fishing pole, whose tip is pulled down by a wriggling ten-pound "minnow." The cervical vertebrae, riding on their disk shock-absorbers, are brought forward to the limits of their flexion capacity, and they stay there. The disks, meanwhile, are under great stress; the muscles of the neck and upper back have locked up from the strain of holding the head's extra weight; lateral and rotational movements can't take place smoothly or even at all. The conditions are in place for a stiff neck, neck pain, and damage to the cervical disks.

Dysfunctional Children: Future Shock

The neck's simplicity, efficiency, and specialization mean that it gets into trouble quickly. It has hardly any extra margin for improvisation and compensation. When the body is fully functional, neck flexion and extension alternate naturally and easily as the load-bearing joints and other structures move in and out of neutral positions. In a typical dysfunction the neck must struggle to climb uphill, lugging the head all the way, in order to achieve a neutral position from which it can accomplish extension. And like Sisyphus, the mythical king condemned to repeatedly roll a boulder to high ground, then see it tumble back down again, the head flops forward when flexion occurs, and the whole grueling process must start all over again. Condemned to live with shoulders hinged forward and hips tilted back, the neck takes the easy way out: It stays at the bottom of the hill, in flexion.

This process is happening earlier and earlier in life. As infants, we create the cervical curve in the spine by learning to lift and move the head from a prone position. That, and that alone, is the purpose of the cervical curve: to hold the head vertically while allowing it to move freely. As children, by rolling around, wiggling, stretching, crawling, and standing, we fashion the lumbar curve. Its job is bipedal locomotion. These two spinal curves are intended to last a lifetime—eighty, ninety, a hundred years, choose a number. Yet today they are beginning to disappear (if they fully form at all) in early adolescence. And that scares the hell out of me.

A few decades ago, a gawky teenager whose head was forward and whose shoulders were slouched was probably showing signs of nothing more than a rapid growth spurt. Before long, the posture muscles would catch up. Today, teenagers still undergo a growth spurt, but it occurs in the context of an increasingly motionless environment that does not provide them with the stimulus they need to awaken and strengthen the supporting musculoskeletal functions. The posture muscles never catch up with the growth spurt. Thus, the head, going along for the ride—remember, it's not the cause of anything—moves forward, not at sixty years old but at sixteen.

We have become so used to seeing heads out of position that it now seems perfectly natural. To see the problem with 20/20 vision, visit a local high school and take a look at hundreds of youngsters in one place. They'll be short or tall, fat or thin, but almost all of them will display signs of major musculoskeletal dysfunction. Fashionable baggy clothes may hide it (and I believe that kids are so uncomfortable with their bodies, they instinctively want clothing to camouflage this vulnerability), but short of wearing a hood, the head cannot be concealed. If you stand in the crowded school hallway as those heads pass by, you'll see pain, depression, anger, illness, boredom, anxiety, and fear on the faces. You'll see the future.

HOW TO GAIN IMPORTANT HEALTH INFORMATION

Put your child up against a wall; and/or put yourself up against it, too. With your shoulder blades touching the surface, is your head touching the wall, too? If you have to pull it back to make contact with the wall, it is positioned forward of the vertical line that should run through the ankles, hips, and shoulders. You are now in possession of important information. It will explain a lot: why you can't get a good night's sleep or are having trouble backing the car out of the driveway; why your child is clumsy or prefers computer games to jumping rope; and why descending stairs, hitting a golf ball, and putting in long hours at a desk reading and writing aren't as easy as they once were. Many routine physical activities depend on a functional head position for their execution. When you have trouble doing them, the wall test will help explain what's going on.

Treatment for Stiff Neck and Neck Pain

In the clinic, the basic treatment we use for stiff necks or neck pain releases the neck from flexion by reengaging the load-bearing joints and posture muscles. Do these E-cises in the order presented.

Total time: Twenty minutes.
Times a day: Once in the morning.
Duration: Do exercises daily until pain abates for forty-eight hours, and then move to the overall conditioning program in chapter 13.

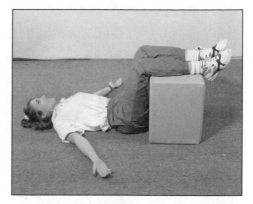

- STATIC BACK

Follow the instructions for
Static Back in chapter 5
(figure 5–5, page 70). Hold
the position for five
minutes. Static Back uses the level floor as a template to bring the
muscles and structures of the body, including the neck and head,
to a neutral position.

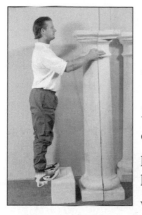

- GRAVITY DROP

Follow the instructions for Gravity Drop in
chapter 9 (figure 9–5, page 157). Hold the
position for three minutes. Gravity Drop the
load-bearing joints in vertical alignment
while statically loaded.

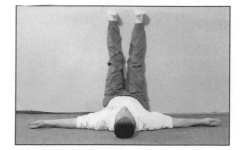

- STATIC WALL

Follow the instructions for
Static Wall in chapter 5

(figure 5–6, page 71). Hold for three to five minutes. This E-cise allows the ankles, knees, and hips to function without being subject to torquing from above by misaligned shoulders.

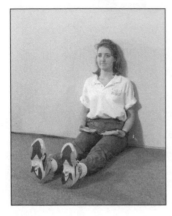

• SITTING FLOOR

Follow the instructions for Sitting Floor in chapter 6 (figure 6–11, page 95). Hold for three to five minutes. Sitting Floor loads the hips and shoulders while reminding the (unloaded or semiloaded) knees and ankles how to operate functionally.

• FROG
  (Figure 11–2)

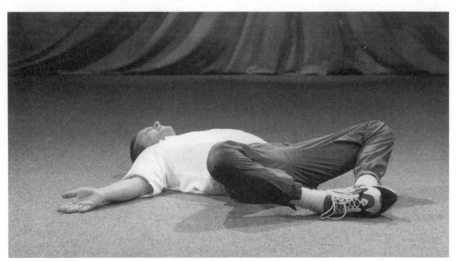

Figure 11–2

Lie on your back, pull your feet toward the torso, and put the soles of your feet together, letting your knees turn out. Make sure your feet are centered in the middle of the body. The low back does not have to be flat on the floor, but you should not feel pain in your back. Don't press down on your knees; relax. You want to feel a comfortable stretch in the inner thighs and groin. Hold for one minute. Frog tames the powerful thigh and groin muscles while putting the pelvis into a neutral position to allow proper flexion and extension.

Spinal Cord Injuries

Whiplash injuries and broken necks are also occurring more frequently because the head has come so far forward that the neck loses its flexibility and shock-absorbing capacity. Hit from behind, the head pops downward, which is exactly the direction it's pointing toward. Since the head is already at or close to the limits of flexion, it has no give; nor does it have the option to recoil smoothly in the opposite direction. Instead, it must make a violent, flopping, pendulumlike movement from front to back, without braking action from the muscles. Consequently, the mechanisms of the neck are traumatized by the impact.

The crash dummies that are used in testing automobile safety equipment give the false impression that whiplash happens when the head reaches the limit of its forward movement and then snaps back. But that's what happens to dummies, not humans. The human head, atop a dysfunctional body, is already at the limit of its forward flexion, and in that situation it has nowhere to go but down. The shoulder yoke, the cervical vertebrae, and the musculature are all driven that way, and the head has no choice but to follow. When it hits the "wall," the uncontrolled bounce back finishes the job.

Effective treatment of whiplash must recognize this situation and be aware that even *after* the accident the head is still forward

---

SPINAL CORD INJURIES

Football players and athletes in other contact sports are experiencing a rise in spinal cord injuries because so many of them come to the game with heads that are forward and out of position. The popularity of weight training makes the situation worse. Lifters bring their heads and shoulders forward and down to execute the move. They do it repeatedly without offering balanced stimulus to other muscle groups. The strengthening muscles lock their heads in this position. Hit from behind, they get badly hurt.

---

and the mechanisms of the neck remain in a position that will continue to cause pain. The object of treatment is to return the body, from head to foot, to vertical alignment, to withdraw it out of the box that it is struggling so hard and so painfully to topple into.

Headaches: What Do They Tell Us?

Suppose you get behind the steering wheel of a car and drive off. You take a quick left, then ask the car to climb a tree, jump over a puddle, or turn a somersault. What will happen? Unless your name is Evel Knievel, the results will be unpleasant and expensive. But we expect our bodies to be able to do all of those things on demand. I think the body's extraordinary prowess leads us to assume that it is not subject to standard operating procedures, aside from the obvious things like feeding it, watering it, resting it, and not running it off a cliff. In a way, we're right: The body has great tolerance. But it does not have infinite tolerance. Unfortunately, many of us need pain to tell us when we've crossed the limits to its tolerance. The pain message, however, is easily garbled. What does a headache, for instance, really mean? Overwork? Hunger? Stress? A brain tumor?

I advocate starting with the most obvious possibility and moving toward the least obvious. For the most part, however, this is not the formula that is used by modern medicine. Its technology allows us to start with the least obvious possibility—on the molecular level, if need be—and work backward; only we never get all the way home to the obvious, because the hardware is not suited to performing on that level. Many clients come to the clinic for headaches and positional vertigo after having undergone extensive testing, including repeated brain scans, all of which have drawn a blank. One woman, Mary Beth, was rarely without either a low-grade headache or a severe migraine. Since nothing showed up on the tests, the doctors here had concluded it was her imagination. She had a low-grade headache when she walked into the clinic.

One of the first things I noticed about Mary Beth was her slightly bulging eyes. That wasn't my imagination, or hers. Nor was her head position a fantasy: It was a good four inches forward of the vertical line that should have run up through the load-bearing joints. Her head position gave us our "most obvious" starting point. We used the E-cises included in this chapter, which are designed to reposition the head, and within ninety minutes she was free of headache for the first time in three years. She did get sick to her stomach, but it didn't last long. Typically a person who's had to contend with a painful condition over long periods of time becomes disoriented when it abates; nausea, dizziness, and acute anxiety are common. It takes a while to get used to being pain free.

Mary Beth's headaches were typical in another way as well. They were a symptom of oxygen starvation. The integrity of the vertical axis through the body is important not only to biomechanical functions like walking, bending over, stretching, and arm movement, but to respiration and circulation. When the thoracic back moves forward into flexion, it restricts the area that the diaphragm muscle under the lungs uses for expansion. Without the diaphragm's help, the lungs cannot fill to capacity. Furthermore, when shoulders—like Mary Beth's—are rolled forward and down, they act to constrict the chest cavity that houses the lungs. Both conditions seriously impede oxygen intake.

Like most people, Mary Beth had never considered that posture has a direct link to brain function. An unstable, semicollapsed musculoskeletal system cannot efficiently perform its role as an oxygen pump. The impediment goes even beyond disrupting the diaphragm and lungs. In a forward head position, the muscles adjacent to the arteries that travel through the neck to the head do not fully assist in the uphill transportation of oxygen-rich blood to the brain. In general, the flexion and extension of muscles help propel blood through the circulatory system. But muscles that are locked in flexion or that are flaccid from disuse cannot do this. It is a major loss of biomechanical capacity. I have never known a migraine sufferer whose head, neck, and shoulders were not out of position in the characteristic mode of forward flexion.

Muscles also allow the eyes to focus and to adjust the amount of light that reaches the photoreceptors of the retinas. These muscles are small and specialized, but like any other muscle, they must have adequate oxygen to operate. As the flow of oxygen diminishes—that is, as the hemoglobin is less and less oxygenated because of biomechanical limitations—the muscles of the eye lose their fine-tuning ability. And the subtlety of adjusting the eye's lens, pupil, and iris makes setting the precision valve we were discussing earlier appear crude and clumsy by comparison. Starved of oxygen, the muscles lose the ability to quickly and smoothly adjust to changes in light levels and focal plane. Like *any* muscle that cannot recharge and re-

THE OXYGEN PUMP

The brain is extremely sensitive to even relatively small fluctuations in oxygen flow. I believe that many of our mood shifts and general feelings of either well-being or anxiety relate to how much oxygen is reaching the brain at any given moment. Even though we live at the bottom of a "sea" of oxygen, it does not simply gush or trickle into our lungs automatically. It must be drawn in and distributed by biomechanical action, another musculoskeletal process that is taken for granted.

juvenate itself, they underreact, overreact, and generally blunder around trying to do the job—and can't. The less oxygen they receive, the worse the problem gets. The migraine sufferer rushes to turn out the lights and to cover his or her eyes with a cold towel. The pain is terrible!

So to treat migraine and other headaches, let's start with the obvious symptoms—and try to restore oxygen flow. Here are four E-cises that work to do so.

> **Total time: Ten minutes.**
> **Times a day: Once in the morning.**
> **Duration: Do exercises daily until pain abates for forty-eight hours, and then move to the overall conditioning program in chapter 13.**

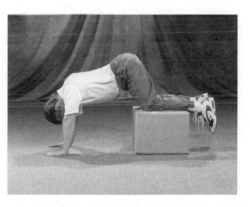

• Static Extension

Follow the instructions for Static Extension in chapter 4 (figure 4–7, page 56). Hold for one minute, building to two minutes. This E-cise unlocks your shoulder blades and the hinge joint of the shoulder, which is stuck in the forward position, to allow the neck to move back into extension.

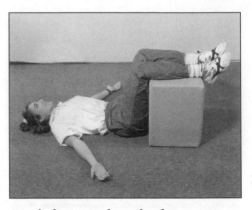

- STATIC BACK

Follow the instructions for
Static Back in chapter 5
(figure 5–5, page 70). Hold
the position for five minutes. Don't forget to breathe from your
diaphragm. Flexion of the thoracic back robs the diaphragm
muscle of operating space. Static Back literally works to give you
breathing room.

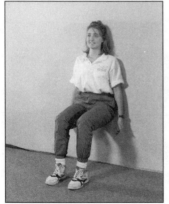

- AIR BENCH

Follow the instructions for Air Bench in
chapter 4 (figure 4–8, page 57). Hold
for one minute, building to two. By
using the power of the ankles and knees, this E-cise convinces the
hips, shoulders, neck, and head that they are capable of operating
in vertical alignment.

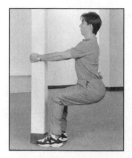

• SQUAT

Follow the instructions for Squat in chapter 8 (figure 8–11, page 136). Hold for one minute. Squat puts the head, neck, shoulders, and hips into proper alignment while loading them equally and engaging the right muscles; by keeping them static, there's no rotation to fight.

Balance: When the Earth Moves

In many cases, poor balance, dizziness, and positional vertigo can also be effectively treated by starting with the most obvious possibility instead of looking for the least obvious symptoms of chronic disease. Once again, the head's position can give us important information. If the head is tipped forward and down, or left to right, what's the most obvious effect? It changes the positions of the eyes, ears, and nose. Our spatial sense—our sense of where we are in relation to where everything else is—functions mostly through our eyes and inner ear. The eyes seek the horizon (or a reasonable facsimile) as a point of orientation. The location of the horizon is more useful for this pur pose than the contours of the ground, which are subject to change. Even as the ground shifts, the horizon remains constant, which allows the brain to send signals to the appropriate muscles to make necessary adjustments to keep the body upright and moving.

Awareness of the horizon, then, lets us know what's up and down, right and left, front and back. This reference point is fixed by three semicircular canals in the inner ear that together function like a carpenter's level, using tiny hair cells set in a gelatinous substance known as the *otolithic membrane.* As we move and our head changes position in relation to the horizon, the force exerted on the hairs by the surrounding membrane changes; they perceive more pressure on one side than the other. The canals project in three different directions at right angles and can therefore detect movement in three dimensions.

When the body is dysfunctional, however, and the head no longer rides level with the horizon, the inner ear canals don't know it. If the head is forward, they assume the body is going downhill, because that's what the pressure shift in the ear canals is reporting. Likewise, if the body has lost bilateral weight distribution, they read it as constantly tipping to the right or left. The eyes, meanwhile, know better; they see the horizon and override the inner ears' signals to the brain. The eyes, in this case, are paramount and take over. Try it yourself: Tip your head to the left while walking in a straight line on level ground. It's hard because the inner ear is telling the brain that you are traversing a steep slope that falls off to the left. You can do it, though, because the eye overrules the inner ear in a conflict. Yet, without the inner ear's help, the eye cannot level the head or the rest of the body. Under these circumstances, balance can be difficult to maintain.

> ### CHECKING YOUR HEAD POSITION
>
> **Stand up straight. Close your eyes, and keep them that way for as long as you can until you start to sway. How long was it? Some people have to open their eyes after only ten or twenty seconds, otherwise they'd fall over. What's happening is that the eyes, when open, are overriding the inner ear's balancing mechanism. Without them, the inner ear takes over and immediately gets confused by the dysfunctional head position.**

Bouts of dizziness occur when the body starts to fatigue from attempting to process the conflicting signals it is getting from the eyes and ears, and from the sheer extra burden of fighting a losing struggle against gravity in a state of misalignment. Reading the terrain becomes increasingly difficult and chancy. Falls are a major health hazard to the elderly and to younger people as well. We blame them on a slippery pavement or on tripping over an obstacle, but often what should have been an embarrassing stumble turns out to be a harmful sprawl because our ability to stay upright has been corrupted. Is it any wonder? Our eyes tell us that we are level and upright, while at the same time the inner ears are saying, "No, look out, you're about to fall over!"

The worst manifestation of this situation is positional vertigo. The eyes are powerful but not all-powerful. The inner ear continues to record the head's position even though the eyes are overriding its messages. The inner ear knows how important to the survival of the body its job really is. When the eyes continually override the inner ears, they perceive that a crisis is shaping up, and they send out increasingly strong signals to get the brain's attention: "Hey, we're going from vertical to horizontal. Do something!" At some point the inner ears have had enough, or the brain finally decides it can't disregard the urgent messages any longer and immobilizes the body before it gets seriously hurt. We go to stand up, but instead we fall down. The inner ears' message is: "You're not going anywhere!"

The process isn't a disease. The otoliths in the otolithic membrane—they're pieces of calcium carbonate, but think of them as the bits of fruit suspended in a Jell-O salad—are leaning on the hairs in the ear canal. In a functional person, the otoliths swish back and forth, right and left, up and down, jostling the hairs to produce an accurate reading of head movement. When the head gets out of position and stays there, however, the otoliths pool up and keep pressing on the hairs until they send the strongest possible alarm to the brain.

Just before I began to write this chapter, one of the nation's wealthiest and most prominent business executives came to my clinic absolutely convinced he had a brain tumor. The reason: He was having bouts of severe positional vertigo. He had undergone weeks of testing, including psychological examinations and major dental work, but none of it came up with an answer. When he called to tell me what was happening, I urged him to get on his private jet and fly to the clinic immediately.

"How long do you think it will take?" he asked. Brain tumor or not, he was still a busy man.

"About an hour," I said.

"An hour! I've had hundreds of hours of treatment for this thing."

"An hour."

In the end, I was wrong. It took a half hour. The man's symptoms disappeared as soon as we repositioned his head.

Does that mean there are no such things as brain tumors, inner ear infections, and the like? No. My point is that by automatically orienting the diagnostic process toward the major pathologies, we too often miss the most obvious and most treatable conditions.

I find that the next four E-cises are effective for positional vertigo symptoms. Bear in mind, though, that like every E-cise menu in this book, this one is just a first-aid measure. There's no substitute for following a full program to restore total musculoskeletal functions, which is at the end of chapter 13.

Total time: Twenty minutes.
Times a day: Once in the morning.
Duration: Do exercises daily until pain abates for forty-eight hours, and then move to the overall conditioning program in chapter 13.

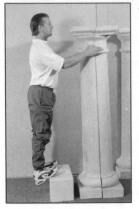

• GRAVITY DROP

Follow the instructions for Gravity Drop in chapter 9 (figure 9–5, page 157). Hold for three minutes. You'll feel your head being pulled back into alignment with the vertical load-bearing joints.

- Static Wall

Follow the instructions for
Static Wall in chapter 5 (figure
5–6, page 71). Hold for three
to five minutes. This E-cise
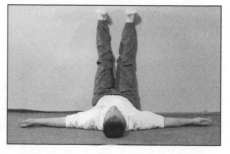
neutralizes the hips, allowing the body, from the waist up and the
waist down, to revert to using forgotten functions.

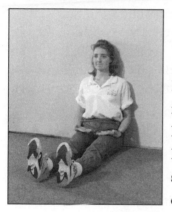

- Sitting Floor

Follow the instructions for Sitting Floor
in chapter 6 (figure 6–11, page 95).
Hold for three to five minutes. Sitting
Floor resumes vertical loading in stages
so that the hips and shoulders aren't in
conflict.

- Static Back

Follow the instructions for
Static Back in chapter 5
(figure 5–5, page 70). Hold
for five minutes. Static Back
isolates the hips, while
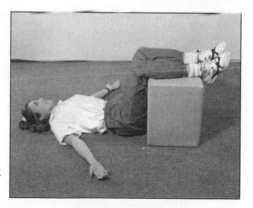
gravity brings the head, neck, and shoulders back where they
belong.

Frequently people come to the clinic for help with one disorder but in the process discover several others they didn't know about. One headache sufferer, for instance, thought his slips and stumbles were nothing more than clumsiness. But as his headaches abated, so did his "bull in the china shop" episodes.

> ## ALLERGIES
>
> Sinuses depend on gravity to drain. Without vertical alignment, this drainage process is interfered with. Congestion is relieved as the head gets pulled back into position. Use the positional vertigo E-cises.

Tinnitus is a condition that often accompanies headaches, poor balance, and positional vertigo. Like the others, its principal effect, ringing in the ears, can be addressed by repositioning the head. The ringing is literally an alarm that is telling us that the inner ear doesn't like the position of the head. If you have that symptom, try the E-cise menu for positional vertigo.

In the Jaws of Pain

The final condition that I will discuss in this chapter is TMJ, or temporomandibular joint dysfunction. The temporomandibular joint is where the mandible—the lower jaw—attaches to the skull. People with severe TMJ can't open their mouths to talk or chew without a great deal of pain. In the worst cases, they can't open them at all. Often, in the early stages, there is a lot of popping and wobbling in the joint as it articulates.

Here again, head position is the key factor. Because the head is flexed forward, the upper torso and neck must recruit muscles to help hold the head in place, muscles that would normally be used to open and close the lower jaw. One theory holds that TMJ is caused when these muscles, which are the musculature of carnivorous predators, overpower the jaw. But our jaw muscles adjusted long ago to not having to tear and crush. Instead, the jaw, and particularly the chin, are unique to a species that uses its mouth to talk more than to chew. But if these muscles are also used for the purpose of keeping the head from flopping over, they tend to go into flexion and stay there. That deprives them of their ability to smoothly articulate the jaw. It gets harder and harder to open one's mouth. Jaw muscles that seem to be tight and overly powerful are actually weak and dysfunctional, forced to choose between opening the lower jaw and letting the head topple forward. The head gets priority.

Here are eight E-cises for TMJ. It is a longer menu than the others, but more muscle groups are involved. Do them in this order.

Total time: Fifteen minutes.
Times a day: Once in the morning.
Duration: Do exercises daily until pain abates for forty-eight hours, and then move to the overall conditioning program in chapter 13.

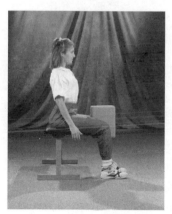

• Sitting Knee Pillow Squeezes

Follow the instructions for this E-cise in chapter 6 (figure 6–10, page 94). Do three sets of twenty; pause between sets. This E-cise strengthens the hip adductor/abductor muscles.

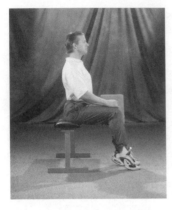

• SITTING HEEL RAISES

Follow the instructions for this E-cise in chapter 6 (figure 6–6, page 90). Do three sets of fifteen. Sitting Heel Raises engage the extensor muscles of the leg.

• STANDING GLUTEAL CONTRACTIONS

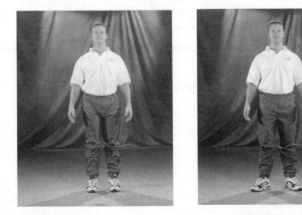

Follow the instructions for this E-cise in chapter 6 (figure 6–5, page 89). Do three sets of fifteen. This E-cise reminds the gluteal muscles that they have a function in flexing the leg.

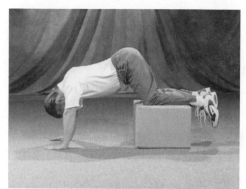

• STATIC EXTENSION

Follow the instructions for this E-cise in chapter 4 (figure 4–7, page 56). Hold for one minute, building to two. This E-cise unlocks the shoulder yokes and neck.

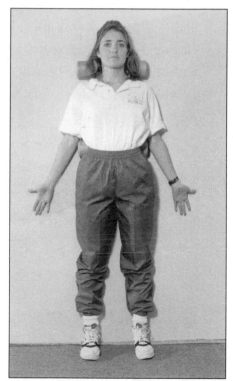

• WALL TOWELS
(Figure 11–3)

Stand with your back against the wall, feet shoulder-width apart and square. Place one three-inch-diameter towel behind the neck and another in the small of the back. Hold for three minutes.

The towels give you vertical support that is otherwise lacking because of the mispositioning of the head.

Figure 11–3

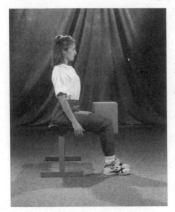

• SITTING KNEE PILLOW SQUEEZES

By repeating this E-cise (the first one on this menu), you are reinforcing the adductors, which are beginning to return to their dysfunctional position at this point in the sequence. Repeat ten times.

• SITTING SCAPULAR CONTRACTIONS

Follow the instructions for this E-cise in chapter 9 (figure 9–3, page 152). Repeat ten times. This E-cise liberates the shoulder blades and reawakens their muscular functions.

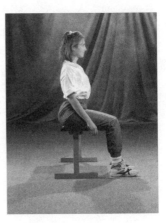

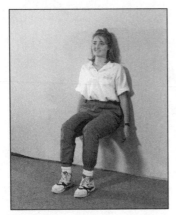

• AIR BENCH

Follow the instructions for this E-cise in chapter 4 (figure 4–8, page 57). Hold for two minutes, building to three. This E-cise puts all the pieces of the puzzle back together again.

To finally bring the elevator to the top floor, let me say that I hope your ascent from foot to head has allowed you to see exactly where you stand—and how.

SPORTS INJURIES AND PEAK PERFORMANCE: PLAY OR PAY

We pay for dysfunctional play with pain—but the price is worth it. Although I'm not an advocate of playing through the pain, the consequences of sidelining oneself are usually far worse than simultaneously pursuing a favorite sport or physical activity and also working to correct the root causes of the pain. This chapter is about the work that must be done to play without pain.

All too often, athletes—be they professionals, dedicated amateurs, or weekend warriors whose field of dreams is a backyard garden or a walk down Main Street—are told that their aches and pains mean that it's time "to go easy." This advice amounts to telling a person lost in the desert and dying of thirst that he needs to drink less water. We are dying of lack of motion. The idea that less motion is the cure is absolute lunacy. Moderation on top of severe motion scarcity leads to a sharp decrease in physical activity. Once an organism reaches crisis, small changes in conditions that would have been insignificant during a period of equilibrium have enormous consequences. For individuals who are living in an environment that provides them with thirty percent or less of the design motion stimulus needed to maintain musculoskeletal health, moderation—a decrease of another five to ten percent—is bordering on a death sentence. I calculate we move on an average of sixty-five to seventy percent less than our great-grandmothers and -grandfathers. It is difficult to quantify exactly, but based on the amount of time modern men, women, and children spend inactive in front of television sets and riding in cars, those two modern "conveniences" alone create a huge motion vacuum.

If our modern lifestyle doesn't provide motion then we have to find other means to obtain this missing essential ingredient. One way—or so we once thought—would be recreation: sports and leisure-time activities to take the place of old-fashioned drudgery. We'd move for the fun of it. Things, however, aren't working out that way.

Golf Is Booming—and Busting

Golf is hot. And it is hot for two reasons: one, people instinctively know they are badly in need of physical activity; two, golf is physically undemanding. But only the first of these reasons is valid. Golf is a demanding sport. But it is also a sport with an image problem. With its white-shoe, country-club aura, it seems the perfect "sport" for those who are sedentary, out of shape, or on the mend from injuries "caused" by other activities. On the contrary, golf requires the athlete to come to the game with balance, strength, and coordination. Without those preconditions, he or she cannot perform well and is likely to get hurt.

A quick review of popular golf magazines and books published thirty and forty years ago turns up only a few occasional references to injuries and how to avoid them. Today, it is a regular theme. Increased health consciousness and the democratization of an elite sport are partial explanations, but clearly more players are in pain and blaming it on golf. The thesis that golf hurts backs has become so pervasive that even the most dedicated golfers, who have never experienced a twinge of pain, believe it to be true. After Tiger Woods joined the pro tour, I received phone calls from journalists wanting to know how long it would be before the young superstar wrecked his back swinging the club as hard as he does. Ironically, Woods will probably end up at some point in his career with back or shoulder problems. Golf will be blamed, even though golf will only serve as the scene of the accident, not its cause.

Woods, like all golfers, didn't get in shape by playing the game, he got in shape by living his life. Sure, his dad had him on the course when others kids were home in front of the TV set. But Tiger did not grow up on another planet. He went through plenty of TV watching, riding in cars, and sitting at desks in classrooms. Like most of his peers, he lacked balanced and complete movement in his daily life. Once he got out on the course, the physical functions he used over and over in practicing the fundamentals did not fill in the gaps in his musculoskeletal functions.

Tiger's right shoulder is forward and lower than the left. This asymmetrical state is evidence of compensation and improvisation. Tiger has recruited muscles and joints on the right side of his body—but not the left—to help him drive a golf ball. The immediate result is a superb athletic achievement. Yet when he leaves the course, those same highly trained and strengthened compensating muscles are doing the mundane work of helping Woods slip on his green Masters jacket, tie his shoes, and sign autographs. Meanwhile, the appropriate muscles and joints on the left side are not participating; there is nothing in the environment, on or off the course, to stimulate them to action. It is this constant imbalance—not the act of hitting a golf ball—that will cause pain if Tiger Woods does not deliberately introduce adequate supplementary motion to replace what he is not getting naturally from his environment.

What's Ahead for a Superstar

In this respect, Tiger Woods is no different from any other weekend hacker. Almost every golfer brings dysfunctions to the game, particularly those who are refugees from more "hazardous" sports. They have the aches and pains that would have occurred even if they had never picked up a club. Increasingly, specific sports are blamed for injuries when those sports may actually be helping the athlete postpone the emergence of the ailment for weeks, months, or years.

In this sedentary culture, any movement is better than no movement at all. The benefits of movement range from continued musculoskeletal stimulation (the absence of which triggers atrophy) to metabolic and cardiovascular conditioning. When we avoid or curtail physical activity, we set in motion a chain of events that leads progressively to disability. It happens very quickly. The benefit of sports—even the so-called hazardous ones—is that they keep the key biomechanical components in motion, to provide strength and support. These benefits would quickly vanish if the athlete retired or took up a less demanding sport that did not fully engage those elements.

> **Less is not more when it comes to motion; less is less. The less you move, the less you are able to move. It's a vicious circle that resembles a noose.**

The Importance of Impact

All of our joints are designed to be loaded and to receive impact. Even when we are sleeping, gravity is pressing down on our musculoskeletal structures. Walking, running, and jumping intensify the load, but that's all right. A functional joint is equipped with rugged mechanisms that help it handle many multiples of the body's total weight as the feet come into contact with the surface of the earth. The eight main load-bearing joints all have muscles that are prime movers and muscles that act as stabilizers during movement. But as our joints become unstable due to misalignment, these mechanisms are corrupted. The stabilizers can't do their jobs completely. When impact occurs, the joint is clobbered in an unstable position. Even so, the stabilizers don't quit entirely. As long as there is loading and impact, they deploy and do their best.

This caveat—"as long as there is loading and impact"—is crucial. The search for low-impact sports and exercise equipment is undermining musculoskeletal function and overall health. I recently saw an ad for a stationary bike-treadmill-skier that suspends the rider in midair using an elaborate frame and stiltlike handles for support. "Your feet never touch the ground," the ad proclaims. The idea is to eliminate all impact. What's happening, though, is that the machine takes an already unstable joint through a range of motion with its stabilizer muscles deliberately switched off. The less impact, the less stabilizer engagement—and the more joint instability. Machines like that one weaken the stabilizer muscles while strengthening the prime movers, to propel an unstable joint through an increased range of motion. This "conditioning" process sends the individual back to the real world to walk, to run—to move—with acutely unstable joints that have been conditioned for a low- or no-impact environment, which doesn't exist short of a coffin.

No matter what the sport or activity, joint instability will take a toll in performance limitations and pain. Swapping your running shoes for a bike, as an example, only serves to change the type of demand that's being put on the unstable mechanisms. It may mask symptoms or postpone the onset of pain, but the dysfunctions are still grinding away.

Golf and tennis are prime examples. Both sports are increasingly being played by the equipment rather than by players. Technological advances in both golf clubs and tennis rackets allow athletes to hit the ball harder and with greater accuracy than was possible just ten years ago. It's easier than ever to get a blistering serve over the net or send a ball straight down a fairway. This improvement in speed, distance, and accuracy has little to do with athletic ability, and nothing at all to do with causing tennis and golf injuries. On the contrary, this fabulous new equipment allows players to do more and more with less and less function. Without the new clubs and rackets, pain symptoms would appear much sooner. Any increase in the number of injuries

> ## CHRONIC PAIN AS A VARSITY LETTER
>
> It used to be that people chose a sport or activity to suit their interests or talent. Increasingly, many of us make the decision based on what works with our dysfunctions. This ends up strengthening the very processes that are causing the chronic pain that we hoped the activity would help us avoid.

in the two sports is solely attributable to the epidemic of musculoskeletal dysfunction that's sweeping through the population as a whole. These are accidents that are waiting to happen—and they happen on golf courses and tennis courts as they do anywhere else.

The Play's the Thing

What follows is an overview of specific popular sports, their problem areas, and E-cise menus for pain symptoms that develop during or after play. If you are experiencing pain, use the appropriate E-cises both before and after the activity. The idea is to move the joints into a neutral position to start and then to reposition them again after they've been moved out of alignment by exertion.

Golf

Going to the driving range is painful, for me. It hurts to see men and women trying to force their frozen shoulders, necks, and heads through the range of motion necessary to get a ball off a tee and into the air. It's not a pretty sight. Musculoskeletal compensation occurs from head to foot. Many golfers suffer from knee, low back, elbow, and shoulder pain. Here are five E-cises that will help relieve those symptoms.

- ARM CIRCLES
  (Figure 12–1 a and b)

Stand with your head up, feet squared, and arms at your sides; put your hands in the golfer's grip, with fingers curled, knuckles flexed, and thumbs extended. Raise your arms out to your sides, keeping your elbows straight, palms down, and thumbs pointing forward (a). Lift your arms until they are level with the shoulders. If one shoulder wants to wobble forward or pop up, lower both until they stay level. Now squeeze the shoulder blades together

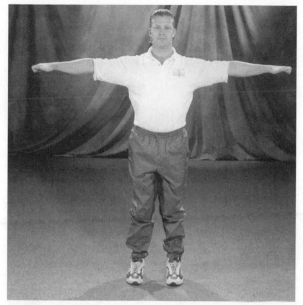

Figure 12–1a

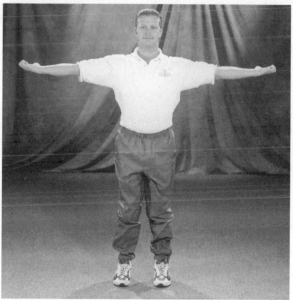

Figure 12–1b

slightly, and rotate the arms forward (in the direction the thumbs are pointing) in a six-inch-diameter circle (b). Do it twenty-five times. Reverse the circles by turning the palms up and thumbs back. Repeat for a total of fifty times in each direction. This E-cise strengthens the muscles of the upper back that are involved in ball-and-socket work.

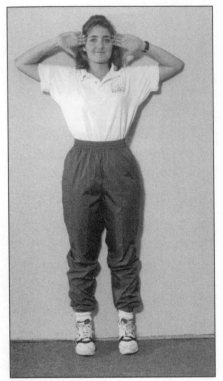

Figure 12–2a

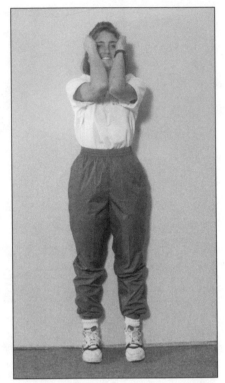

Figure 12–2b

- ELBOW CURLS
  (Figure 12–2 a and b)

Using both hands and the golfer's grip (see Arm Circles), raise
them palm-out so that the flat area between the first and second
knuckle joints of the index and middle fingers rests on the
temples in front of the ears; the thumbs are extended downward,
parallel with the cheeks. Draw the elbows back evenly and in line
with the shoulders (a). From this starting position, slowly swing
the elbows forward until they touch in front (b). Keep the
knuckles in contact with the temples, the thumbs fully extended,
and the head erect. If the head moves back and forth, stand up

against a wall, slow down, and breathe deeply. Do twenty-five Elbow Curls.

This E-cise is a reminder to the shoulder that it has a hinge function.

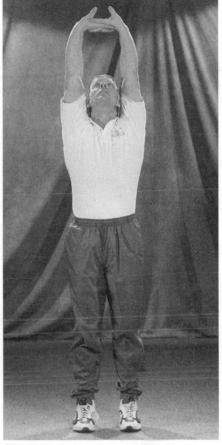

• Standing Overhead Extension
(Figure 12–3)

Stand with your feet straight, hip-width apart. Interlace your fingers, rolling the palms toward the ceiling, extending the arms overhead with elbows straight. Look up at the backs of your

Figure 12–3

hands. Work on keeping the arms in vertical alignment with the shoulders and the rest of the body. Hold for one minute.

This E-cise points all the load-bearing joints in the right direction and engages the neck.

- UPPER SPINAL FLOOR TWIST
  (Figure 12–4)

Lie on your side with your knees bent, to form a right angle to the trunk. Extend both arms along the floor level with the shoulders, keeping the elbows straight with the palms together and parallel with the bent legs. Slowly lift the upper arm up and over to rest behind you on the floor palm-up while you turn your head to face the ceiling. Adjust this arm position, if necessary, by finding a shoulder slot that's comfortable, while relaxing and breathing deeply. Allow gravity to settle the arm to the floor along its entire length from fingers to shoulder. Meanwhile, make sure the knees don't slide apart. You can hold them in place with the other hand (as the model is doing). When the shoulders have leveled out right to left (it may take several minutes and perhaps several sessions to achieve this fully), lift the extended arm and return it to the starting position while exhaling. Repeat on the other side. This E-cise puts both shoulders and arms on the same plane.

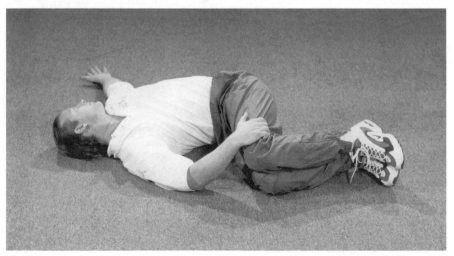

Figure 12–4

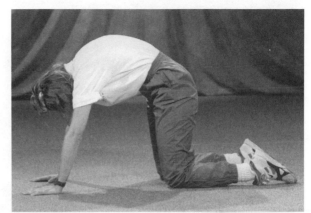

Figure 12–5a

- CATS AND DOGS
  (Figure 12–5 a and b)

Get down on the floor on your hands and knees. Make sure your knees are aligned with your hips and your wrists with your shoulders. Your lower legs should be parallel with each other and with the hips. Make sure your weight is distributed evenly. Smoothly round your back upward as your head curls under to create a curve that runs from the buttocks to the neck—this is the cat with an arched back (a). Smoothly sway the back down while bringing the head up—this is the perky dog (b). Make these two moves flow continuously back and forth rather than keeping them distinct and choppy. Do one set of ten. This E-cise works the hips, spine, shoulders, and neck in coordinated flexion-extension.

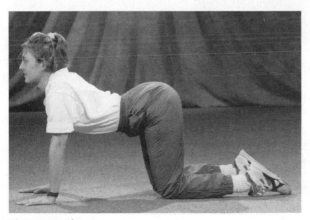

Figure 12–5b

Tennis/Racquet Sports/Handball

Tennis, the other racquet sports, and handball are regarded as hard on wrists, elbows, and shoulders, but they're not. The extra demand of playing those games merely pushes already dysfunctional players over an edge they would eventually encounter at home or at the office anyway. Here are five E-cises that address the source of wrist, elbow, and shoulder pain.

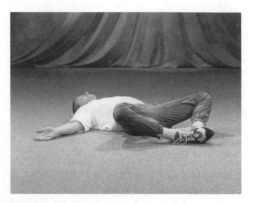

• FROG

Follow the instructions for Frog in chapter 11 (figure 11–2, page 194). Hold for one minute. This E-cise puts the hip into a neutral, bilateral position.

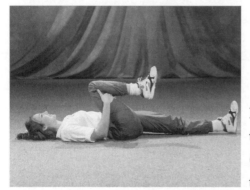

• FOOT CIRCLES AND POINT FLEXES

Follow the instructions for this E-cise in chapter 4 (figure 4–5, page 53). Do twenty circles each way, building to forty. Then do ten point flexes, building to twenty. This E-cise gives the foot, ankle, and calf muscles a wake-up call so that they will operate in a heel-ball-toe gait-pattern.

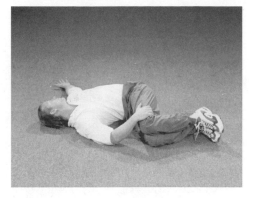

• UPPER SPINAL FLOOR TWIST

Follow the instructions for this E-cise in the golf section of this chapter (figure 12–4, page 220).

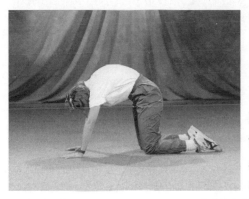

• CATS AND DOGS

Follow the instructions for this E-cise in the golf section of this chapter (figure 12–5 a and b, page 221).

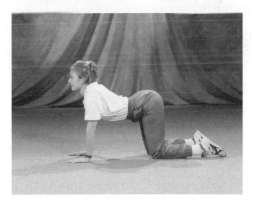

- DOWNWARD DOG
  (Figure 12–6 a and b)

Assume the Cats and Dogs position (a). Curl your toes under, and push with your legs to raise the torso until you are off your knees and your weight is being supported by your hands and feet. Keep pushing until your hips are higher than your shoulders and have formed a tight, stable triangle. Your knees should be straight, your calves and thighs tight (b). Don't let the feet flare outward; keep them pointing straight ahead in line with the hands, which need to stay in place—no creeping! The back should be flat, not bowed, as the hips push up and back into the heels. Breathe. If you cannot bring your heels flat onto the floor, do what you can to narrow the gap while keeping the legs tight. Don't force them. Hold for one minute. It may take several days or weeks to get the heels flat.

Downward Dog reestablishes linkage from your wrists to your feet.

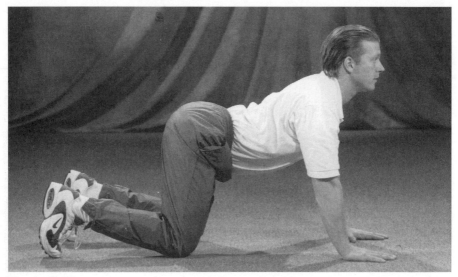

Figure 12–6a

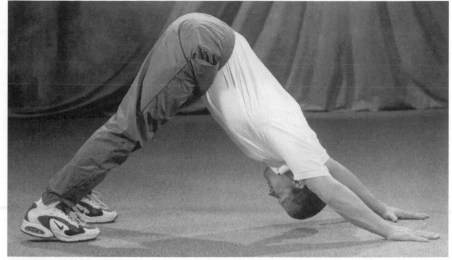

Figure 12–6b

Rowing/Kayaking

Rowing isn't dangerous, but it is endangered. Individuals whose shoulders are rounded forward—most of the U.S. population—are not likely to take up rowing or stick with it for very long. A dedicated rower may retain more shoulder, elbow, and wrist functions than a nonrower does, but even with rowers those functions are often incomplete. In a shell, where the rower is pulling on a single oar, the activity is unilateral; the functions are not being balanced. The situation is different in a single, but in both cases each stroke is strengthening a forward head position and spinal flexion. Kayakers are in the same boat, so to speak. Here are four E-cises for the most common pain symptoms.

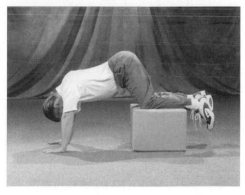

• STATIC EXTENSION

Follow the instructions for Static Extension in chapter 4 (figure 4–7, page 56).

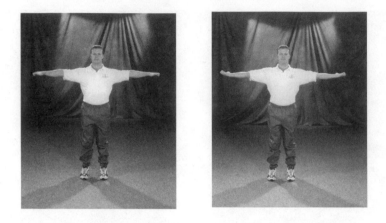

- ARM CIRCLES

Follow the instructions for Arm Circles in the golf section of this chapter (figure 12–1 a and b, page 216).

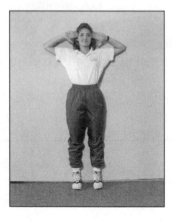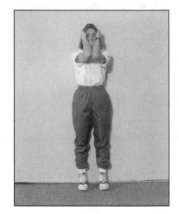

- ELBOW CURLS

Follow the instructions for Elbow Curls in the golf section of this chapter (figure 12–2 a and b, page 218).

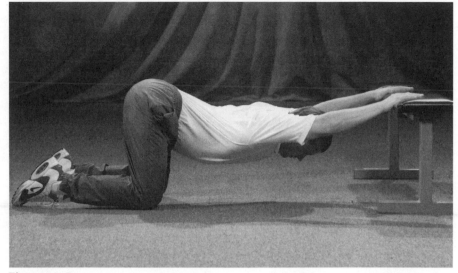

Figure 12–7

- KNEELING COUNTER STRETCH
  (Figure 12–7)

Kneel with your hips over your knees while extending your arms palm-down on a chair or low table. Relax the trunk so the back seems as if it's trying to fall through between the arms. Breathe deeply. Hold for one minute.

This E-cise allows spinal flexion to intervene between the hips and the shoulders.

Ice Skating

TV has fallen in love with figure skating, but the sport itself is not one that attracts huge numbers of participants. At one time, in the colder parts of the country, ice skating was a popular activity, probably on the order of snowmobiling today. But sports that require balance—and ice skating is one of them—lose their following when people are no longer able to smoothly transfer weight from hip to hip. Skaters use their adductor and abductor muscles, reinforcing the strength of those muscles and encouraging them to take

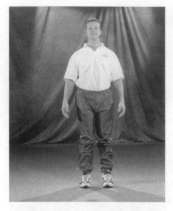

over the normal gait-pattern when walking. As for injuries, skaters tend to have ankle, knee, back, and shoulder problems. I recommend this menu of E-cises.

• STANDING GLUTEAL CONTRACTIONS

Follow the instructions for this E-cise in chapter 6 (figure 6–5 a and b, page 89).

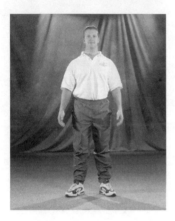

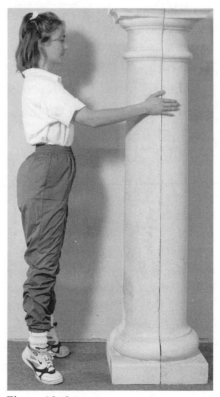

• THREE-POSITION TOE RAISES
(Figure 12–8 a, b, and c)

One: Near a closed door or wall, stand with your feet pointed straight ahead, hip-width apart, with the weight distributed evenly between them. Turn your toes outward

Figure 12–8a

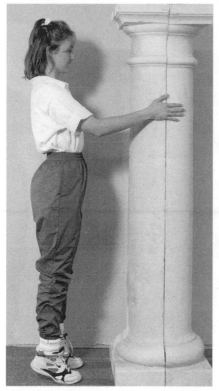

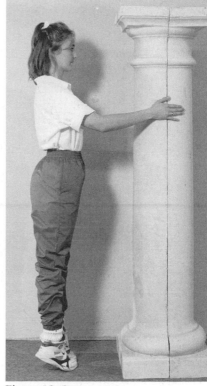

Figure 12–8b   Figure 12–8c

to forty-five degrees. Slowly raise and lower yourself on your toes, keeping your weight equalized on both feet (a). Do ten repetitions. Use the door or wall as a visual guide to vertical alignment so that you are not leaning or lunging forward as you execute the toe raises. *Two:* Keep the same position, but bring your feet parallel, keeping them hip-width apart. Raise and lower yourself on your toes, keeping the weight distributed equally on both feet (b). Do ten repetitions. *Three:* Keep the same position, but angle the toes inward by about twenty degrees. Raise and lower yourself on your toes, keeping the weight equalized on both feet (c). Do ten repetitions. Each of these positions uses a different set and sequence of muscles.

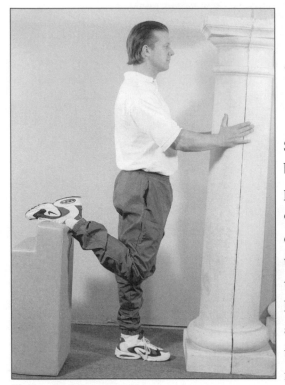

Figure 12–9

- STANDING QUAD
  STRETCH
  (Figure 12–9)

Stand on one foot and bend the other leg back, placing the top of the foot on a block or the back of a chair. The height dictates the amount of stretch in the quadriceps. Keep your hips and shoulders square and your knees even, and tuck your hips under to feel the stretch. If necessary, hold on to something for balance. Hold for one minute, then repeat on the other side.

Hip rotation shuts the quads off; this E-cise turns them back on.

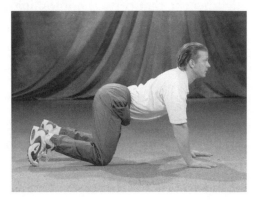

- DOWNWARD DOG

Follow the instructions in the tennis section of this chapter (figure 12–6 a and b, page 224).

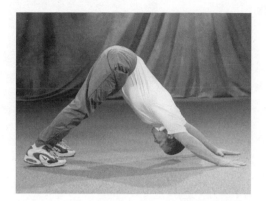

Downhill Skiing/Cross-Country/Snowboarding

The modern ski boot puts the skier's hips, legs, knees, and ankles into the extension position, which is where they are supposed to be to control a pair of skis. The problem is that most skiers are already in flexion because of their dysfunctions. This situation produces enormous stress on joints that are unstable to begin with. To relieve chronic knee pain, use these E-cises.

• SITTING KNEE PILLOW SQUEEZES

Follow the instructions for this E-cise in chapter 6 (figure 6–10, page 94).

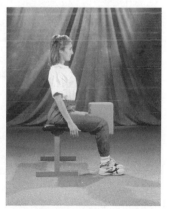

- STATIC EXTENSION
  (POSITION)

Follow the instructions for
Static Extension in chapter
4 (figure 4–7, page 56), but
perform it on the floor
rather than up on a block.

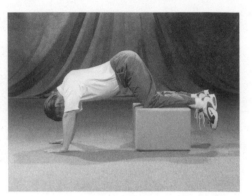

- CATS AND DOGS

Follow the instructions for Cats and Dogs in the golf section of
this chapter (figure 12–5 a and b, page 221).

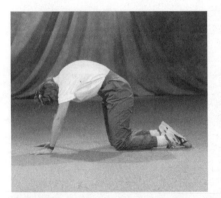 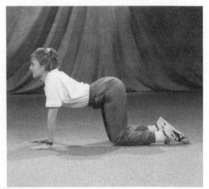

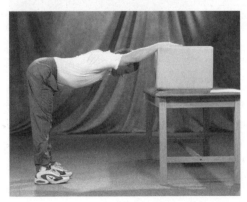

- COUNTER STRETCH

Follow the instructions for
Counter Stretch in chapter
7 (figure 7–4, page 112).

• FLOOR BLOCK

Follow the instructions for
Floor Block in chapter 8
(figure 8–10 a, b, and c,
page 133).

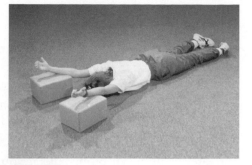

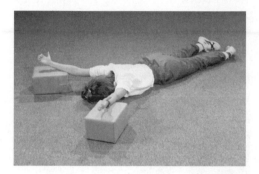

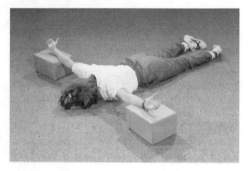

Those who do cross-country skiing don't have the same equipment considerations, but in many cases they are propelling themselves with rotated knees, displaced hips, and backs that are in
flexion. And while snowboarders let gravity provide propulsion,
they have similar dysfunctions. Both should do the E-cises for ice
skating.

Running

Running gets the worst rap of any major sport, and many of its loudest critics are former runners. Their primary objection to running is its impact on the load-bearing joints. When those joints are unstable and out of alignment, their capacity to manage the shock of each foot strike is indeed impaired. Fancy shoes and knee braces won't help, nor will adjustments in technique. These E-cises will mitigate the pain symptoms, but if you're a runner and want to remain with the sport, you'll have to work on restoring lost functions by using the E-cises in the next chapter.

• DOWNWARD DOG

See instructions for Downward Dog in the tennis section of this chapter (figure 12–6 a and b, page 224).

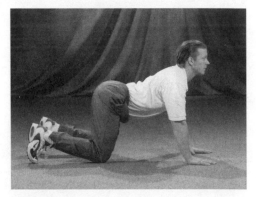

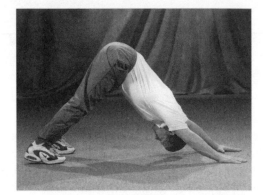

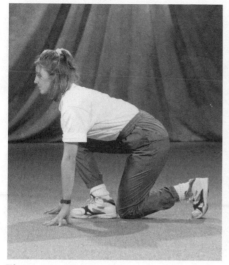

Figure 12–10a

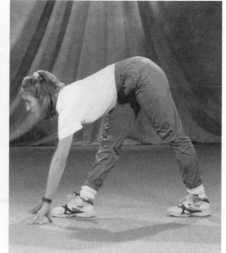

Figure 12–10b

- RUNNER'S STRETCH
  (Figure 12–10 a and b)

Kneel on one knee. With the other leg, place the heel of the foot in front of the knee that is on the floor. The heel and knee should make contact slightly. For balance, rest your hands on the floor or on a chair or block placed just in front of the forwardmost foot (a). Curl the toes of the back foot under and stand up on both feet (b). Your hips should be square, heels down, and both legs straight. Contract the thigh of the front leg as you position the upper body so that it moves over the front foot and leg. You should feel a stretch along the back of the forward leg. Keep the upper body relaxed as you hold the stretch for one minute. Release the stretch by kneeling back down into the starting position. Reverse the legs and repeat. This E-cise is reminding your muscles and joints that when the left side of the pelvis flexes, the right extends (and vice versa). At first, you'll probably find that it is easier to do on one side than the other.

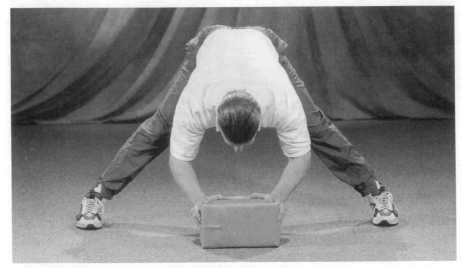

Figure 12–11a

- SPREAD FOOT FORWARD BEND
  (Figure 12–11 a, b, and c)

Stand with your legs spread wide. Keep your feet pointed straight ahead. Bend over at the hips and touch the floor directly in front of you. If that's too difficult, you may use a block, book, or other prop for support. Tighten your thighs and relax your torso toward the floor (a). Hold this position for one minute. Next, without straightening up again, slide your hands to your right foot (move the prop, if you're using one), keeping both thighs tight and the torso relaxed (b). Hold that position for one minute. Then, slide left to the center briefly before moving your hands to the left foot (c). Again, keep your thighs tight and your torso loose. Hold for one minute. Finally, move to the center, bend your knees, and roll your torso upright. This E-cise puts your hips into a neutral position and allows your prime movers to do their jobs without the secondary muscles getting in the way.

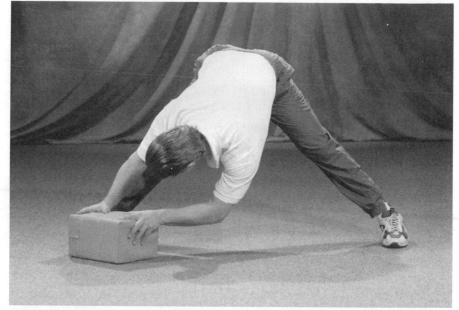

Figure 12–11b

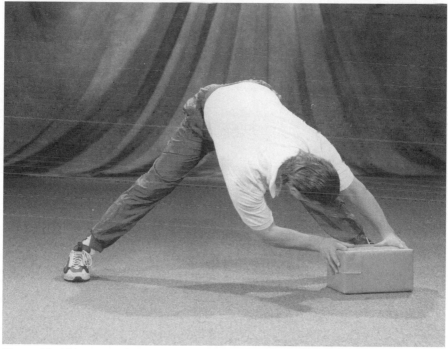

Figure 12–11c

Cycling

Cycling is a favorite refuge of former runners. In fact, some running gurus recommend alternating biking with running to give the body's joints an opportunity to recover from the pounding. But for someone with misaligned joints, all cycling does is postpone the onset of pain. An unstable but rested joint is still unstable. Cyclists avoid impact, but they send their misaligned joints through a repeated range of motion for mile after mile. The activity also reinforces flexion and hip problems that are characteristic of people who sit for most of the day. The appeal of many sports and physical activities is often based on how directly the motion required is linked to the dysfunctional motion of the athlete's daily life. Cyclists feel comfortable in the saddle because it approximates the sitting position they are in for most of their waking lives; even the forward head position and the downward roll of the shoulders are familiar. If you have pain in the knees, hips, back, or shoulders, try these E-cises.

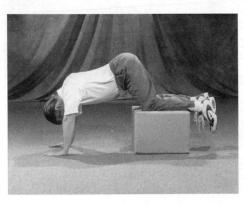

• STATIC EXTENSION

Follow the instructions for Static Extension in chapter 4 (figure 4–7, page 56).

• DOWNWARD DOG

Follow the instructions for Downward Dog in the tennis section of this chapter (figure 12–6 a and b, page 224).

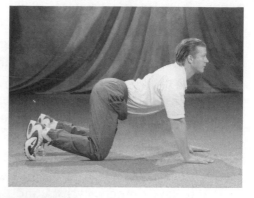

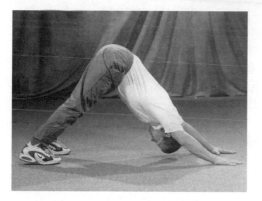

• SQUAT

Follow the instructions for Squat in chapter 8 (figure 8–11, page 136).

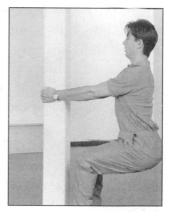

Walking

Walking (or swimming) is often the runner's last resort. Walking is being heavily promoted these days as an effective and benign form of exercise. And it is effective. Walking is great, and not an activity to be regarded as suitable only for the elderly or those recuperating from surgery and cardiac incidents. If you're walking with a dysfunctional body, however, walking is going to ask you to pay with pain. The impact is less than running, but the joints still receive shock. An unstable joint will eventually react, much to the surprise of those who believe that walking is "exercise lite." If you are a walker and have joint pain, follow the E-cise menu I laid out for runners.

In-Line Skating

These days runners, cyclists, and walkers are sharing the same space with in-line skaters. There's a natural dysfunctional affinity among these activities, and my guess is that many in-line skaters are former runners and cyclists. In-line skating has far less impact than running, and you can cover more ground with less ankle, knee, and hip involvement. Both considerations are important to people whose locomotion is primarily being handled by the rotator muscles of the hip, the muscles of the low back, and the shoulders. Also, in-line skating caters to everted feet; that's the position the foot assumes to achieve the semilateral thrust of the skate's blade. This posture brings the head and shoulders forward for balance. Impact injuries, which are on the rise, are usually in the wrist and knee, which are sticking out and waiting to be whacked. Generally, chronic pain symptoms for in-line skaters are focused in the shoulders, low back, and knees. Try the E-cises for ice skating.

Swimming

Swimming is often one of the last stops for runners and walkers (and in time probably for in-line skaters, too) because there is no impact. But even without impact, a dysfunctional swimmer can experience pain. Just taking unstable and misaligned joints through a range of motion is enough. Forward flexion of the hips and torso—the modern posture—doesn't go away because the athlete is in water. Swimmers can experience neck, shoulder, and back pain. If you have such a problem, these E-cises will help.

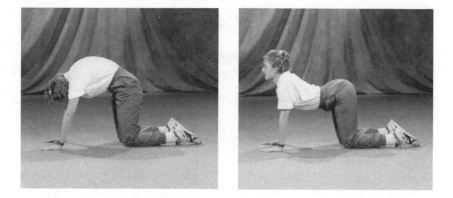

• CATS AND DOGS

Follow the instructions for Cats and Dogs in the golf section of
this chapter (figure 12–5 a and b, page 221).

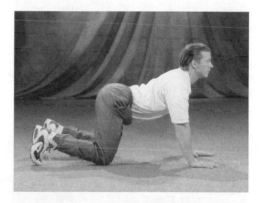

• DOWNWARD DOG

Follow the instructions for
Downward Dog in the
tennis section of this
chapter (figure 12–6 a and
b, page 224).

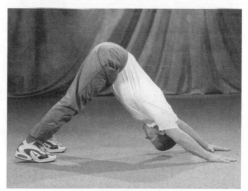

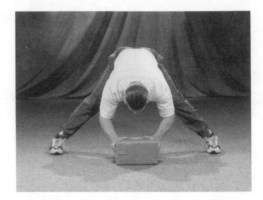

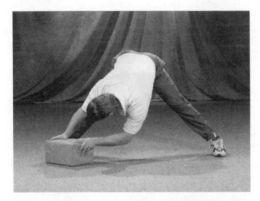

• SPREAD FOOT
FORWARD BEND

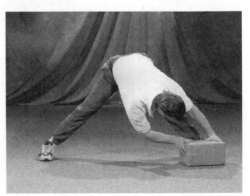

Follow the instructions for
this E-cise in the running
section of this chapter
(figure 12–11 a, b, and c,
page 236).

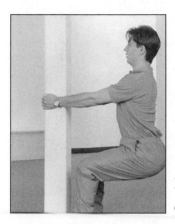

• SQUAT

Follow the instructions for Squat in chapter 8 (figure 8–11, page 136).

Gymnastics

Gymnasts impress everybody with their amazing flexibility, so it's easy to mistakenly conclude that their flexibility equals fitness. But many of these athletes start working at an early age on extending the range of motion of their joints without developing underlying strength and stability. The result is a hypermobile joint that is subject to damage because it is operating on the far edge of its range of motion without an adequate muscular foundation. Particularly among men, the peripheral torso muscles are impressive and well-defined, but the deep posture muscles tend not to be properly developed enough to avoid injury. For load-bearing-joint pain, try the following menu of E-cises.

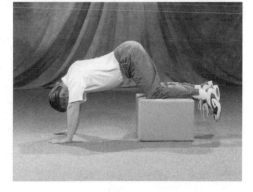

• STATIC EXTENSION

Follow the instructions for Static Extension in chapter 4 (figure 4–7, page 56).

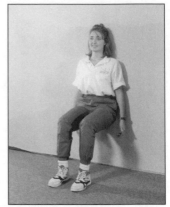

- AIR BENCH

Follow the instructions for Air Bench in chapter 4 (figure 4–8, page 57).

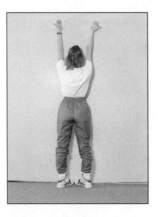

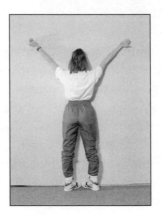

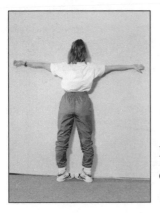

- WALL CLOCK

Follow the instructions for Wall Clock in chapter 10 (figure 10–5 a , b, and c, page 173).

• DOWNWARD DOG

Follow the instructions for Downward Dog in the tennis section of this chapter (figure 12–6 a and b, page 224).

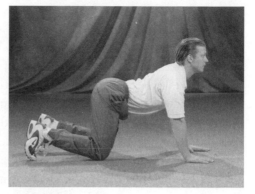

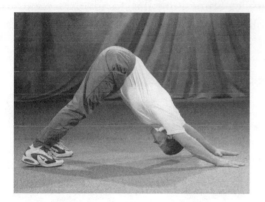

• SQUAT

Follow the instructions for Squat in chapter 8 (figure 8–11, page 136).

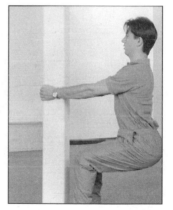

Weight Training

I enjoy weight training, but I've learned to keep my mouth shut in the weight room. Many weight lifters are their own worst enemies. They work hundreds of hours to strengthen their musculoskeletal dysfunctions. Most dedicated athletes tend to work the hardest on muscles and structures that are, one, the strongest to begin with and, two, the most accessible. This means that the surface and peripheral muscles get the bulk of the attention and the deep muscles are neglected. Unfortunately, dysfunction sets in from the inside and works outward. The deep muscles, large and small, go first. Function is transferred to the next layer up, until finally most of the work is being done on the surface. These muscles are the survivors; they hang on because they are able to improvise the means to operate unstable joints. Weight training strengthens that capacity. The result is an unstable joint being driven by a stronger and stronger compensating muscle. Something has to give. Here are E-cises that weight lifters will find useful.

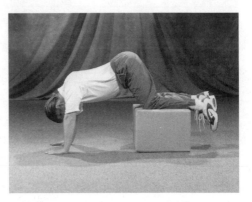

• STATIC EXTENSION

Follow the instructions for Static Extension in chapter 4 (figure 4–7, page 56); hold for two minutes.

• CATS AND DOGS

Follow the instructions for Cats and Dogs in the golf section of this chapter (figure 12–5 a and b, page 221); do fifteen of them.

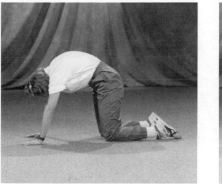
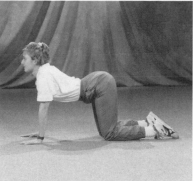

• DOWNWARD DOG

Follow the instructions for
Downward Dog in the
tennis section of this
chapter (figure 12–6 a and
b, page 224); hold for one
minute.

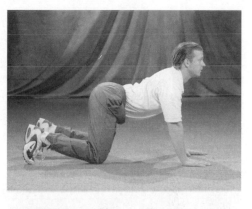

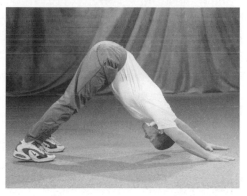

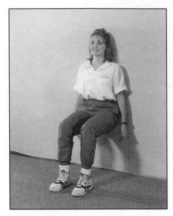

• AIR BENCH

Follow the instructions for Air Bench in chapter 4 (figure 4–8, page 57); hold for two minutes.

Soccer

The American public is finally discovering soccer. It is an excellent sport. The growing interest in participation is being fueled by the perception that traditional team sports like football, baseball, and basketball are either too hazardous, too physically demanding, or too body-type determinate (that is, by bulk, strength, or height). As a running game, soccer is making use of the modern body's sturdiest structures—the hips and legs—and assigning a much smaller role to the weaker, dysfunctional upper body. Much to the delight of soccer moms and dads, the potential for injuries doesn't seem as great, but that's largely a misperception. World-class soccer is a rough-and-tumble contact sport that has its share of mayhem. Kids love the game because it gives them a chance to run, kick, duck, dodge, twist, and turn—motion that they instinctively want but aren't getting in their daily lives. But this is also where the problems arise: Saturday-morning soccer is not going to make up for a week's worth of motion starvation. Knee and back pain do occur. Here's a set of E-cises for those pain symptoms.

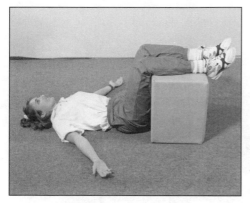

• Static Back

Follow the instructions for Static Back in chapter 5 (figure 5–5, page 70).

• Abdominal Crunchies
(Figure 12–12 a and b)

Lie on the floor and place your feet on the wall, with knees bent, hip-width apart (a). Your feet should be straight and parallel. Clasp your hands behind your head, with the elbows held level

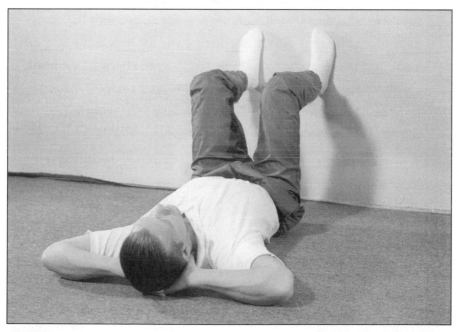

Figure 12–12a

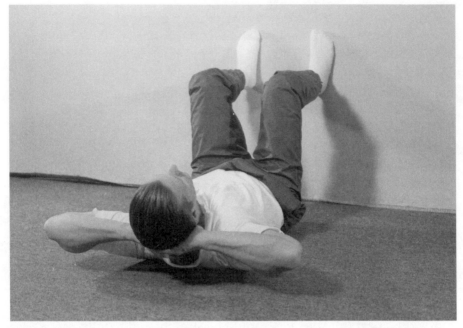

Figure 12–12b

with the floor. Don't pull on the neck to lift the head; rather, allow the arms, shoulders, neck, and head to lift as one unit (b). Keep your face looking at the ceiling during the lift. When the line of sight breaks eye contact, it is time to lower the back to the floor. Do three sets of fifteen. Relax a moment after each set.

This E-cise forces your abdominals to do the work rather than the hip flexors or the thoracic back muscles.

• STATIC EXTENSION (POSITION)

See the instructions for this E-cise under Downhill Skiing in this chapter (page 232).

- SETTLE ON TOWELS

Use two rolled towels, approximately three and a half inches in diameter. Lie flat on the floor on your back. Place one towel under the small of your back, just above the waist, and the other under your neck (not under the head). Breathe deeply, and hold for three minutes.

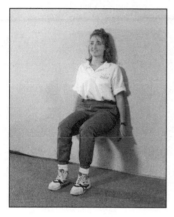

- AIR BENCH

Follow the instructions in chapter 4 (figure 4–8, page 57).

Volleyball

The popularity of volleyball parallels the soccer paradigm, then reverses it. Like soccer, volleyball appeals to those seeking a noncontact team sport that isn't dominated by power players. Also, it has a relative amount of equality between the sexes. But unlike soccer, volleyball makes heavy use of upper body functions, which quickly start showing pain symptoms, primarily in the shoulders, elbows, and wrists. The need to transfer weight quickly also catches up to the back, knees, and ankles. If you are a volleyball player and have such symptoms, use these E-cises.

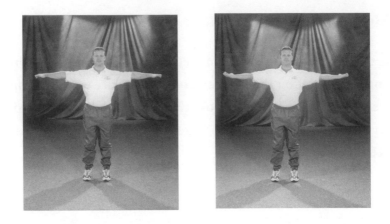

- ARM CIRCLES

Follow the instructions for Arm Circles in the golf section of this chapter (figure 12–1 a and b, page 216).

- SITTING FLOOR TWIST
  (Figure 12–13)

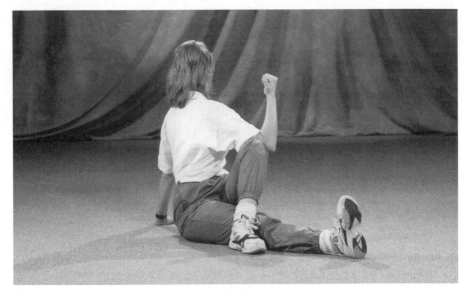

Figure 12–13

Sit on the floor with your legs extended in front. Bend your left leg, and cross it over the right. Keep the left foot flat on the floor and running parallel to the right leg. Place the right elbow outside the left knee, twisting the torso to the left. Your head is now facing behind you. Tighten the muscles of the straight leg, and flex the ankle back toward the knee. This E-cise forces the hip rotators to behave bilaterally and to function in cooperation with the shoulders. Breathe. Hold for one minute, then repeat on the other side.

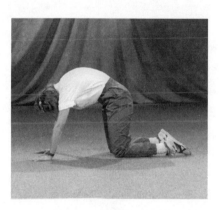

• CATS AND DOGS

Follow the instructions for Cats and Dogs in the golf section of this chapter (figure 12–5 a and b, page 221).

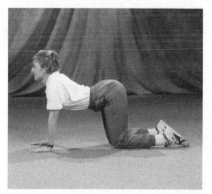

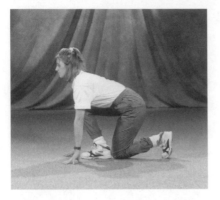

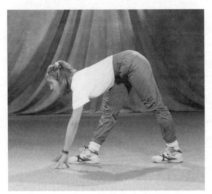

• RUNNER'S STRETCH

Follow the instructions for
Runner's Stretch in the running
section of this chapter (figure
12–10 a and b, page 235).

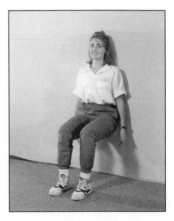

• AIR BENCH

Follow the instructions for Air Bench
in chapter 4 (figure 4–8, page 57).

Baseball

Recently I was listening to a major-league game on the radio when a collision at second base knocked the wind out of the runner. One of the sportscasters dryly observed, "Well, if you play this game, you can expect to get hurt." What? Are we talking about baseball, that game where one player pitches a ball, another hits it with a bat, and, if he succeeds, a third tries to catch it?

Baseball was not always perceived as a bruising sport, but in recent years its injury rate has grown amazingly high. The reason is not that today's athletes are playing the game harder than their predecessors; rather, they are playing with more dysfunctional bodies. A functional musculoskeletal structure can take the shock of sliding into second base, but a dysfunctional one can't. The same goes for pitchers, whose load-bearing joints are out of alignment as they attempt to deliver ninety-mile-an-hour fastballs again and again. Dysfunction is the reason for the rash of shoulder injuries, sore arms, and bad backs among pitchers, even though most of them rarely play all nine innings but are specialists who relieve, close, or hold on defensively to a lead. Pitchers of Dizzy Dean's generation did it all, and they did it in back-to-back doubleheaders.

Here are E-cises for typical baseball pain symptoms.

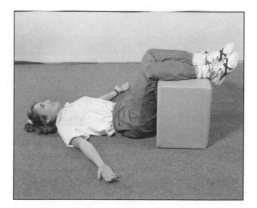

• STATIC BACK

Follow the instructions for Static Back in chapter 5 (figure 5–5, page 70).

- ABDOMINAL CRUNCHIES

Follow the instructions for Abdominal Crunchies in the soccer section of this chapter (figure 12–12 a and b, page 249).

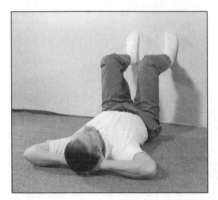 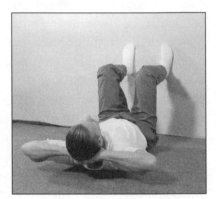

- CATS AND DOGS

Follow the instructions for Cats and Dogs in the golf section of this chapter (figure 12–5 a and b, page 221).

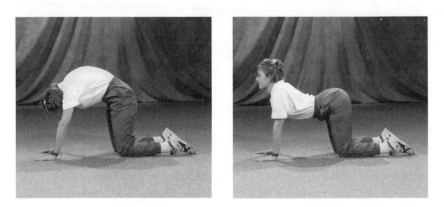

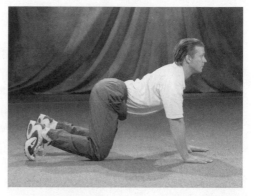

• DOWNWARD DOG

Follow the instructions for
Downward Dog in the
tennis section of this
chapter (figure 12–6 a and
b, page 224).

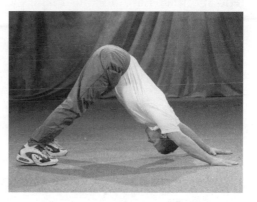

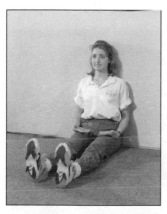

• AIR BENCH

Follow the instructions for Air Bench in
chapter 4 (figure 4–8, page 57).

Football

    I was a college player with a full athletic scholarship, but I'm
afraid football has started to bore me, and it gets worse with every
season. Coaches and players are attempting to do with bulk and

strength what was once primarily accomplished with athletic skill, stamina, and finesse. Today's typical players find it difficult to change direction, which certainly limits what they can do on the field. Their difficulty is caused by the hip misalignment that athletes bring to the game. Without kinetic linkage among all the load-bearing joints, they are also vulnerable to serious injury when they change direction or get hit. Knee problems are now so routine that the sports press has convinced the public that knees are humankind's weakest anatomical mechanism. These commentators imply that knees must be inherently fragile if such magnificent athletic specimens are hurting them so often. On the contrary, the problem is that football players have weight-trained and conditioned themselves into worse shape than many an average nonathlete of the same age.

These E-cises work for football pain symptoms.

- Kneeling Groin Stretch
  (Figure 12–14)

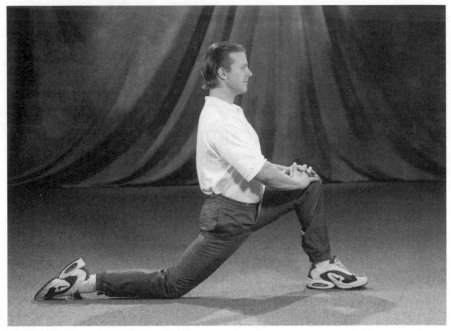

Figure 12–14

From a kneeling position, place one foot out in front of the other with the knee bent. With the head up and the back straight, place your interlaced hands palm-down on the front knee, and lunge forward. Keep your hips square, and avoid twisting the trunk. Do not let the front knee move beyond the ankle. Hold for one minute, then repeat on the other side.

You should feel this E-cise in the groin. It reminds the groin muscles that their job is to help stabilize the hip.

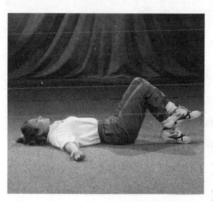

- ISOLATED HIP FLEXOR LIFTS ON A TOWEL

Follow the instructions for this E-cise in chapter 6 (figure 6–7, page 91).

- HAND/LEG OPPOSITES BLOCKED (Figure 12–15)

Lie on your stomach with your arms straight overhead. Place a six-inch block under one arm, with its lower edge two inches from the elbow (toward the wrist). Place another six-inch block under the opposite leg, with the upper edge two inches above the knee (so as to avoid kneecap discomfort). Rest your forehead on the

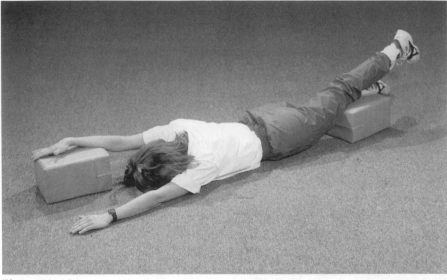

Figure 12–15

floor. Let the stomach settle into the floor as the shoulders and buttocks relax. Hold for three minutes. Switch sides and repeat.

This E-cise counteracts dysfunctions that affect the smooth interaction between transversely opposed limbs.

- CATS AND DOGS

Follow the instructions for Cats and Dogs in the golf section of this chapter (figure 12–5 a and b, page 221).

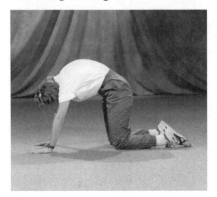
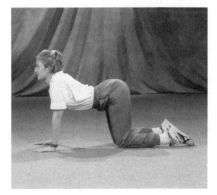

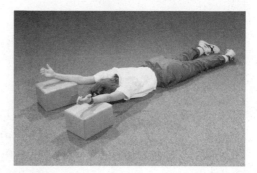

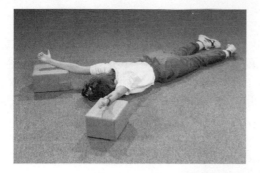

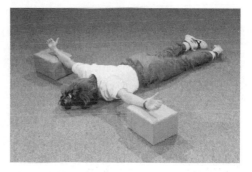

• FLOOR BLOCK

Follow the instructions for Floor Block in chapter 8 (figure 8–10 a, b, and c, page 133).

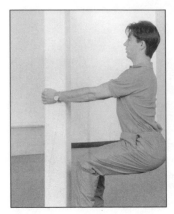

• SQUAT

Follow the instructions for Squat in chapter 8 (figure 8–11, page 136).

Basketball

I'm impatient with basketball, too. The game gets cruder and more violent with every season. Scoring in the NBA is way down, primarily because shooting skills are deteriorating as players lose their shoulder functions. A shoulder that is rolled forward and down cannot bring the arm into a full vertical position over the head. Thus, players take shots from unstable compensating positions. They know it, so instead of shooting from outside, they want to bring the ball to the basket so they can stuff it. That's why there's so much contact and fouling. Players' ability to sink free throws has become abysmal, along with offensive team play that requires a spatial sense of what's going on and the ability to respond in coordination with one's teammates. Knee, back, and shoulder injuries are common. This set of E-cises will help with the pain symptoms— but not the poor playing.

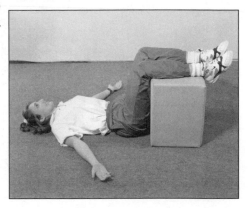

• STATIC BACK

Follow the instructions for Static Back in chapter 5 (figure 5–5, page 70).

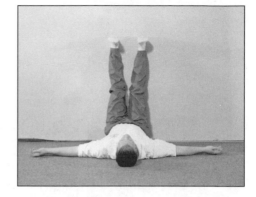

- STATIC WALL

Follow the instructions for
Static Wall in chapter 5
(figure 5–6, page 71).

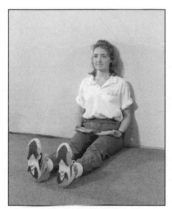

- SITTING FLOOR

Follow the instructions for Sitting Floor
in chapter 6 (figure 6–11, page 95).

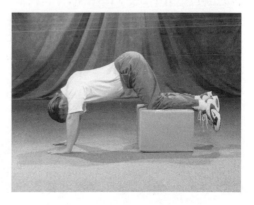

- STATIC EXTENSION

Follow the instructions for
Static Extension in chapter
4 (figure 4–7, page 56).

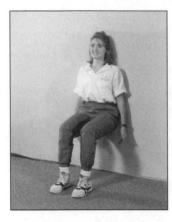

• AIR BENCH

Follow the instructions for Air Bench in chapter 4 (figure 4–8, page 57).

Health Clubs

I've saved this one for last because health clubs and fitness centers are great ideas, and those who use them don't deserve to have bad things happen. I'll focus briefly here on why these establishments don't fulfill their promise.

The trouble starts with limited motion and then it continues with limited motion. Fitness-center apparatuses and the routines they foster are isolating only a few muscles and structures. They make no attempt to balance the stimulus. The typical individual goes into the health club already out of balance, then usually proceeds to work on structures that are already the strongest and hence the most gratifying. He or she naturally wants to see progress. Compensating muscles, rather than dormant prime movers, respond the most readily to such workouts, because they are engaged and active.

The StairMaster is a great example. People spend hours on the machines strengthening the peripheral muscles that rotate their hips. The flexor-extensors—the hamstrings, glutes, and quads—are neglected. But those are precisely the muscles that get flabby and need the work.

Ever hear of StairMaster Butt? It's a term I picked up from a *Washington Post* article that noted the phenomenon, especially among women, of ballooning backsides despite heavy workouts on the StairMaster and similar machines. What's happening is this: The work is strengthening the peripheral muscles, which bulk up and push outward on the atrophied gluteal muscles. This produces a ballooning effect rather than a slimming one.

Even if you do manage to isolate and exercise specific muscles with health club equipment, the moment you dismount the muscles disengage and return to their dormant state. For the rest of the day, these muscles are out of it. The other problem with isolating muscles is that these muscles don't perform musculoskeletal functions in isolation. By picking and choosing to strengthen some muscles and to ignore others, structural imbalance is guaranteed. This is definitely the case with all the popular ab machines that are being sold today. Their greatest sin, as far as I'm concerned, is taking backs that are already in flexion and conditioning the muscles to keep them there.

Finally, the low-impact/no-impact obsession has swept through health clubs and fitness centers. Aerobic dancing and other high-impact aerobic routines are now almost nonexistent, and that's a shame. There is simply no such thing as a stable joint that is not under load and not subjected to impact. High-impact aerobics serves that purpose well.

If you are a health club member with pain symptoms, consult the chapter that deals with the specific body part that's involved.

To close this chapter, I want to reemphasize that none of these sports, activities, or pieces of equipment causes pain. The motion they provide is better than nothing. The only game we need to quit playing is the blame game. It is our responsibility to find the way back to a life of motion.

13

PAIN FREE:
THE RIGHT
TO MOVE

Now that you have alleviated your pain by using the E-cises in chapters 4 through 12, you may be wondering how to stay pain free. This chapter takes you beyond first aid to what I call Ultra Aid—a lifetime program to defeat chronic pain.

A Little Motion Goes a Long Way

There is nothing wrong with first aid; indeed, it is essential to survival. Modern Western medicine is very good at first aid, at dealing with traumatic, life-threatening events. But this adeptness of ours has led to the creation of a crisis context for health care in which established treatments are largely elaborate and often drastic first aid techniques. These are sometimes appropriate, but not on a routine basis. For one thing, the human musculoskeletal system has its own built-in first aid system for dealing with most problems. All we need is an understanding of its basic operating principles and a willingness to do our part to support them. Don't worry, I'm not proposing a "buns of steel" approach to fitness and health. What I'm proposing begins with getting more motion into our lives. I suggest keeping a motion diary, log, or journal. It could look something like this:

MORNING

Hour 1   Woke up, showered, dressed, made breakfast, drove the kids to school.

Hour 2   Drove to work, answered phone messages.

Hour 3   Attended meeting, reviewed annual-report draft.

Hour 4   Interviewed job applicant, made calls, had lunch at desk.

AFTERNOON

Hour 5   Meeting—boring!

Hour 6   Cab to client's office, discussed problems and prospects.

Hour 7   Cab back to my office, answered phone message, drafted memo.

Hour 8   Conferred with Ronnie and Alice, went through the mail.

Hour 9   Drove to the grocery store, shopped, drove home.

EVENING

Hour 10   Prepared dinner, ate, did cleanup.

Hour 11   Drove to choir practice, practiced.

Hour 12   More choir practice.

Hour 13   Drove home, helped kids with homework.

Hour 14   Did office paperwork, checked the computer for E-mail.

Hour 15   Watched TV, got ready for bed, went to bed.

This diary may not come anywhere near your normal routine. It's just a template that you can customize in order to track your motion for a couple of weeks, until you begin to see patterns. That's the key word, *patterns*. Modern life imposes a distinct pattern on why and how we move. Patterns become so routine we are no longer aware of them. The diary technique will make your pattern visible so that you can see your hourly, daily, and weekly motion. What you can see, you can change.

After a few weeks of keeping the motion diary, do a motion analysis. Make a rough estimate of how much time you spend driving, sitting at a desk, and watching TV. When you are moving, what are you doing, and what parts of the body are participating? Do you primarily walk short distances? Do you use your hands at waist level? Do you extend one arm again and again? This information is all valuable because it shows us not only what we are doing but what we are not doing. It is that data that will allow us to change the pattern.

Most people would say that they are constantly moving, and that's probably true. But they are constantly moving only a few parts of their bodies. The human body has 187 joints and more than 600 muscles, and all of them must move or they will quickly lose function. This rule even applies to nonlever joints like those that connect the bones of the rib cage and the vertebrae of the spine. But if I sat down and dreamed up a program to consciously move every one of those joints and muscles at least once a day, I would end up with a routine that would take hours and hours to fulfill. Not even the most dedicated fitness fanatic could do it. Fortunately, there's no need for it. A fitness routine that can handle the job already exists: life. Many muscles are involuntary, like the heart. There's no need to consciously send its muscles a signal to produce the desired response. The rest of the muscles are voluntary. But they'd just as soon go about their business without a great deal of conscious second-guessing. These prime and secondary movers are the ones that are susceptible to patterned motion for the simple reason that before the modern era, wide variation of movement was the pattern. Now it isn't.

If your motion diary tells you your motion pattern is dictating movements that primarily involve the hands and elbows, you'll know that your shoulders, among other structures, need something to do. The diary will also show you what parts of your body are clocking up hours of activity and those that are putting in only minutes. The more a musculoskeletal structure is used, the stronger it gets. This explains why our bodies lose balance and bilateral function. A five-minute walk to the bathroom and back every couple of hours is not going to fully counteract the strengthening that occurs when we ask certain muscles and joints to hold us in a sitting position for five or six hours. Yet if we are aware of this time and motion disparity, we can do something about it.

Do what? Add one nonpatterned movement each hour. If you are sitting down, stand up; if the work is in front, reach behind; if your hands are busy, give your feet something to do by going for a quick walk.

There are dozens of possibilities. Doing one every hour isn't asking for much in terms of time and effort, but it will provide substantial benefits. By deliberately engaging otherwise neglected functions, we strengthen them and boost all the systems of the body.

Many exercise programs make the mistake of asking people to go too far, too fast. The pain and exertion the novice experiences overwhelm the gain. By breaking your entrenched motion pattern only once an hour, you are gaining the capacity and, most importantly, the inclination to break out more often. It becomes fun and self-reinforcing.

> ## PATTERNED MOTION BUSTERS
>
> - **Reach over your head with both hands.**
> - **Twist laterally at the waist.**
> - **Turn your head all the way to the right and left.**
> - **Look at the ceiling.**
> - **Sit on the floor.**
> - **Kneel.**
> - **Flap your arms like a bird.**
> - **Stand on a chair.**
> - **Balance on one leg.**

When I visit major cities, I'm struck by how smokers cluster on downtown sidewalks by the entrances to office buildings, puffing on cigarettes. They've been driven outdoors by no-smoking rules. Ironically, their nicotine addiction is forcing them to disrupt their patterned motion and get up from the desk, go downstairs, and stand around for five or ten minutes. It's easily the one and only benefit to be gained from the habit. But they are also establishing an interesting precedent, and if nonsmokers aren't getting the same privileges, they are being penalized. What I would like to see, on behalf of workplace safety, is a policy that encourages similar patterned motion breaks for everyone. If smokers can do it, so should the rest of us!

A Wonderful Life

I'm often asked to recommend the ideal job or lifestyle for avoiding musculoskeletal pain and dysfunction. That's easy—all of them.

Your body's design is capable of allowing you to be a ditchdigger or a bank manager with equal facility. If the laborer's only physical activity is using a shovel, he or she will be just as dysfunctional as the office worker. Aside from Third World sweatshops ringed by barbed wire and armed guards, I can't think of any occupation that requires workers to stand exactly in the same spot and repeat the same motions every second of every hour. We aren't machines, and we do have latitude to change the pattern enough to give the body the variety it needs to maintain musculoskeletal health.

> It's not what you do at work, but what you do *around* the work that you do.

People with ideal occupations and lifestyles create those circumstances themselves. Recently, I stopped to watch a residential roofing crew on the job. Four men spent the morning climbing up and down ladders and hunching over a roof, hammering nails into shingles. At lunch, they came down and stretched out in the grass to eat sandwiches. They changed their pattern. Then they changed it again: They spent the next half hour tossing around a small football in an impromptu game. They ran, dodged, threw passes, and reached high in the air to snag the ball. They worked hard on the roof, played hard on the ground, and had a great day. Another example of motion variation is set by a friend of mine who never parks her car in the same place when she goes to work. One day she finds a spot at the bottom of a steep hill that she'll have to ascend and descend; on another she stops a mile away to get in a good, brisk walk; and on a third she leaves the car at the edge of a park and jogs the rest of the way in. Sometimes the car stays in the garage while she takes the train. Each situation uses slightly different functions (including those involved in hoisting her heavy briefcase into the train's overhead rack).

Not long ago a woman in her early seventies came to the clinic. She had been a dancer in her youth, and she was still in marvelous condition. Everyone immediately noticed the beauty of her legs. Elaine explained her "secret": While she wasn't dancing any longer, she made sure that at work she only used the ladies' room one floor down from her office. Several times a day, she took the stairs down and back up. That's all she needed to break the pattern. We can all do the same thing. Instead of allowing motionless patterns to be imposed on us, we can devise our own motion-rich patterns.

For a change, children can be the role models for adults, since kids are instinctive pattern busters. Ask a boy or girl to pick

> **MORE PATTERN BUSTERS**
>
> - Carry your suitcase instead of wheeling it.
> - Get out of the car and open the garage door instead of using the remote control. (I won't even bother to suggest losing the TV channel-surfing gizmo.)
> - Put the telephone someplace where you will need to stand and walk to answer it.

up a book that's been dropped on the floor in the dining room. The youngster may wiggle under the table to get it instead of walking around. Children can do the simplest things in the most round-about ways, because they're aware of their own physical nature. They don't try to live apart from it the way adults do. It's not a question of growing up. I think it comes down to not growing at all. If you make proper and regular use of your physical functions, they will continue to increase in capacity. Our adult patterns of motion become fixed and limited probably because we become specialists—moms, dads, CEOs, whatever—and certain roles seem to come with certain patterns of movement. An aide to Robert Kennedy once joked that RFK was so used to traveling with an entourage of syco-phants wherever he went that he had forgotten how to operate a doorknob. It was an exaggeration, but just opening a door is useful motion. Any time physical input is limited, growth stops. In due course, pain begins.

How Lack of Sleep Is Connected to Pain

Motion energizes all of our systems, while lack of motion drains them. In place of motion, we use artificial stimulants—nicotine, caffeine, sugar, alcohol—to manage output and outcome: to get up, to get mellow, to find motivation, to go to sleep. The person with the ideal occupation or lifestyle is one who is using motion as an upper, a downer, and a sleeping pill. The clients who come to my clinic with the worst chronic pain symptoms are also often showing symptoms of acute sleep deprivation. They are irritable, anxious, unfocused, and uncoordinated. The pain is not, I'm convinced, what's causing them to lose sleep. Lack of sleep preceded the pain. It is a result of patterned motion that does not engage the muscles enough to produce fatigue. As muscles lose function, their fatigue threshold rises. They have less need for sleep to reenergize tissue that isn't expending much energy in the first place. This pattern quickly becomes a vicious circle of motion deprivation leading to sleep deprivation causing more motion deprivation the next day and so on. All the body's systems suffer.

Patterns breed their own subpatterns. By moving the fatigue threshold, a pattern of restricted motion leads to staying up late at night—we tell ourselves that we're night owls—to having a nightcap to help relax, a midnight snack because we're bored, lonely, or depressed, or taking pills to make us drowsy. Another pattern within a pattern is poor nutrition and hydration. We use food and drink to replace the lost motion stimulus. If John feels lousy at 10:00 P.M. and eats an extra-large pizza all by himself, are his obesity and crazed blood sugar the result of poor willpower, a rotten job, bad genes, or lack of motion? I vote for the lack of motion. Remember my one-to-ten formula for diagnosis? Start with one, the simple possibility, before you go to ten and get complicated. This is true of hydration, as well. Start with water. Muscle tissue is more than ninety percent fluid. If the fluids ingested are being used to substitute for lost stimulus, we drink coffee, tea, cola, sugary drinks, and alcohol. The muscles are in double jeopardy: Already losing function because of motion deprivation, they are not getting adequate fluid because stimulation occurs sooner than

---

DRINK IT DOWN, FUEL IT UP

- Always serve water with meals.
- Drink a glass of water first thing in the morning.
- Declare water-only zones, such as the bedroom and the car.
- Keep a water bottle or carafe on your desk.
- Substitute fruit juice mixed with sparkling water for soft drinks and sports drinks.
- Replace coffee, tea, or soft drinks with water one day a week.
- When you're dragging, try water first; you may not need anything else.

---

does proper rehydration. The Coke wets our whistle but doesn't refill our fluid reservoirs.

These patterns need to be busted, too. As you track your motion, keep tabs on what you eat and drink as well. Add it to the diary. You will notice that on days when your physical activity is highest, your intake of food and beverages changes in quality and quantity. Artificial stimulation won't be as necessary. But on a cold, gloomy day that keeps you inside and inactive, you will run for the sweets, salt, and coffee. For people with the ideal job and lifestyle, food is for refueling the body, not for stimulation. And they drink water heavily. On the rocks, straight up, fizzy, and still, the brand is H_2O. How much water? Your body will tell you according to how much motion is occurring. Bust the pattern of motionlessness, and you will immediately see your demand for water rising. There's no such thing as too much water.

Beware of Repetition

Believe it or not, exercise itself can fall into motion-limiting patterns. Habits and routines—other terms for patterns—are tech-

niques for managing scarcity. We manage our money; we manage
our time; we manage our energy. As our lives are drained of motion, our ability to respond physically to the environment departs
with it. Consequently, we develop the habit of "unwinding" in
front of the TV, watching sports instead of playing them, and driving the car instead of walking a few blocks. Laziness isn't the issue; the issue is dwindling functions. Exercise is limiting our
motion most when it becomes repetitive: when we follow the same
jogging route day after day, use the same machines at the health
club, ride a bike, and nothing else. Repetitive motion may mean
that you are exercising your dysfunctions, the ones that overpower
the functions and give you just enough oomph to break into a
sweat. Staying in the comfort zone locks you into the zone of dysfunction.

TRANSFORM EXERCISE INTO MOTION-CISE

- Run and walk at different speeds along varied routes.
- Vary the time of day that you exercise.
- Work on the four halves of the body: right half, left half,
  top half, and bottom half.
- Spend some time on *all* the machines in the health club.
- Identify the piece of equipment or routine you hate, and
  use it once a week.
- Vary the impact, demand, and stimulus of the machines.
- Enjoy exercise quickies, and make time for slowies.
- Exercise with different partners.
- Change the environment, the terrain, the temperature.
- Get up off the ground; get down on the ground.
- Take off your shoes.
- Turn off artificial soundtracks—like TVs, audiotapes, and
  radios. The body has its own rhythms that are being lost
  and supplanted by the noise.
- Keep aerobics in perspective: If you do nothing but
  strengthen the heart, you are deconditioning the rest of
  your body.

FUNCTION RUNS

1. **Keep your pace barely over walking speed.**
2. **Loosen up your torso, shoulders, arms, and neck.**
3. **Breathe from the diaphragm.**
4. **Lean back at the waist until you feel perfectly erect.**
5. **Put bounce into your feet, ankles, and knees.**
6. **Let your arms pump easily as you run—left, right, left—but don't let them rise higher than your waist, and keep them swinging straight ahead.**
7. **Concentrate on the heel-ball-toe foot strike, with the feet pointing straight ahead.**
8. **Shoulders back, head up. Look around. Enjoy!**

Sweat is the holy water of exercise, but occasionally it's a good idea to perspire in moderation. At the clinic we hold conditioning camps for professional and amateur athletes, where I introduce them to "function runs." These runs require less moisture and more design function from them. Runners often rack up a fast pace and many miles using compensating muscles and unstable joints. Here's how to avoid the danger in eight easy steps:

Function runs, which can vary a jogging routine by breaking the pattern, are available to almost anyone looking to restore motion to their life. The length may range from twenty minutes to two hours or more. The value of the function run is that it deliberately equalizes your stronger compensating muscles and your weaker prime movers. When we are dysfunctional, heavy exertion demand automatically accesses our strongest muscles. Function runs are a way to stop that from happening and to give those prime movers a workout so they can gain strength.

Let's disrupt one more pattern and then move on to a few final items. Most of us have a habit of saving our breath—managing oxygen. We do it for the same reason that we manage other functions: Oxygen is in short supply. Like fluid intake, air intake is limited by musculoskeletal dysfunction. And again a vicious circle emerges: the less function, the less oxygen; the less oxygen, the less function. We can, however, turn the vicious circle into a virtuous circle. Let's stop saving our breath.

Molecules, Muscles, and Motion = Metabolism

As we break our motion patterns, we are also altering a metabolic pattern that has synchronized itself with our other dysfunctional patterns. One can hardly expect to lose weight, deliver peak mental and physical performance, and experience a sense of well-being if the metabolic rate is dragging.

Understanding metabolism isn't easy, and I'm only going to skim across the surface in explaining how it relates to motion. Metabolism is a process by which the body breaks molecules down into forms of energy. Oxygen consumption is a universal measure of metabolic rate (BMR) because oxygen—oxygenation—must be present for the molecules to come apart, or burn. The only means of delivering oxygen to the body is via the muscles. If muscles don't operate the lungs, we are out of business. But more than mere "air" is

---

TAKE BREATHING BREAKS

- Stand and wiggle your shoulders and neck to loosen them.
- Relax your stomach muscles (a shocking, unchic idea!).
- Close your mouth, and inhale deeply through the nose. Fill the lungs. Engage the diaphragm.
- Don't hold your breath. Exhale through the mouth.
- Inhale and exhale slowly like this ten times.
- Inhale once more. Hold the air in your lungs and slowly count to ten, then exhale.
- Do this routine after rising in the morning, before exercising, and before going to sleep at night (and any other time you feel like it).

involved. A host of chemical reactions drives every bodily process. Muscles, in addition to delivering oxygen, are central to utilizing the energy that is created. This metabolic product is shipped out either in the form of heat or as work. The work has the further advantage of supplying more oxygen. Sixty percent of our body weight is accounted for by muscle and bone. The reason is that we are designed to move, to work—a lot! Metabolism depends on this movement. Muscles and bones, pulleys and levers, put the whole machine in gear and keep it running. When we bring the machine to a halt in a nearly motionless environment, metabolism still goes on—if there's enough oxygen. But the lack of musculoskeletal work profoundly disrupts the ongoing chemical processes of the body. We weaken, get sick, and die.

A Final Set of E-cises

This final series of E-cises will help to counteract your slide into dysfunction and pain and provide a foundation upon which a full restoration of functions can eventually be built. If you are coming directly from a bout of chronic pain, which you have suppressed with the appropriate E-cises, phase in this menu by doing it three times a week for a month. After that you can do it daily. If the chronic pain returns, go back to the original menu until it is gone.

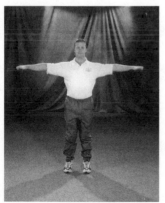

• ARM CIRCLES

Follow the instructions for Arm Circles in chapter 12 (figure 12–1 a and b, page 216). This E-cise is deceptively simple and fiendishly difficult for some people.

Do it in front of a mirror to see if both
arms are on the same level. If they're
not, adjust them until they are. Do fifty
repetitions. The upper back muscles are
getting a good workout in collaboration
with the shoulders.

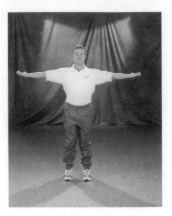

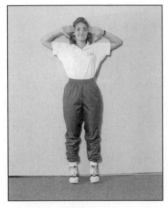

• ELBOW CURLS

Follow the instructions for Elbow Curls
in chapter 12 (figure 12–2 a and b, page
218). Do fifteen Curls. Every good
hinge must move forward *and* back.

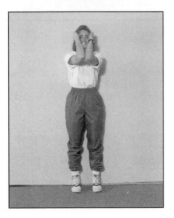

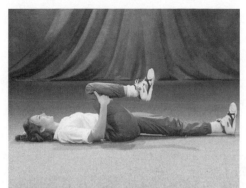

• FOOT CIRCLES AND
POINT FLEXES

Follow the instructions for
this E-cise in chapter 4
(figure 4–5 a and b, page 53). Do twenty of each, on both sides.
This simple one is also tough for people who usually walk like
ducks, with their feet everted.

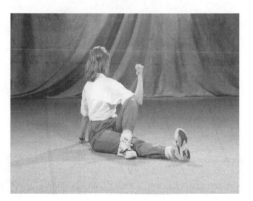

• SITTING FLOOR TWIST

Follow the instructions for
this E-cise in chapter 12
(figure 12–13, page 252). It is difficult in direct proportion to the
loss of bilateral function in the hips and shoulders. You'll know
it's working when both sides start feeling the same. Hold for one
minute on both sides.

• CATS AND DOGS

Follow the instructions for Cats and Dogs in chapter 12 (figure
12–5 a and b, page 221). Do one set of fifteen. This E-cise runs a
flexion-extension drill for the hips, spine, and shoulders.

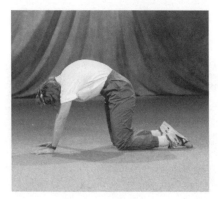
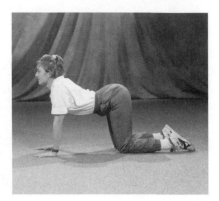

• KNEELING GROIN STRETCH

Follow the instructions for this
E-cise in chapter 12 (figure
12–14, page 258). Hold for one
minute, and repeat on the other
side. This E-cise reminds the

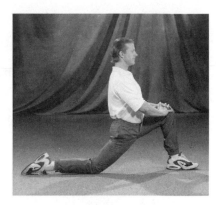

groin muscles that they are not primary hip flexor-extensor
muscles.

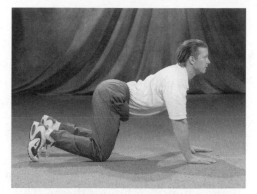

• DOWNWARD DOG

Follow the instructions for Downward Dog in chapter 12 (figure 12–6 a and b, page 224). Hold for one minute. This E-cise recruits all the posterior muscles instead of just a few of the more powerful ones.

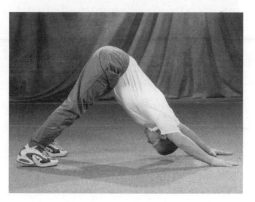

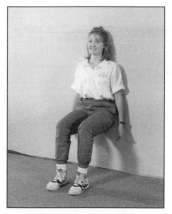

• AIR BENCH

Follow the instructions in chapter 4 (figure 4–8, page 57). Hold the position for two minutes, building to three. Thigh muscles enjoy sitting down so much, they forget that they're supposed to help with supporting the trunk; this E-cise is a little reminder.

I recommend you do this routine daily, in the order it is presented. Once again, if you feel pain, it's a message that your dysfunctions are still in control. Turn back to the appropriate pain chapter and do those E-cises until it abates.

From First Aid to Ultra Aid

I titled my first book *The Egoscue Method of Health Through Motion.* It was a pretty ambitious theme. This one, *Pain Free,* is more modest. Each uses a different route to get to the same place: the realization that thanks to our marvelous musculoskeletal heritage, we all have the power to control our own health and to live pain free. But just having power isn't enough. Power must be exercised. Fundamentally, to preserve and protect what makes us uniquely human, it is necessary to fight for the right to move.

NOTES

Chapter One

For general myological and human physiological data and definitions used in this chapter and throughout the book:

John Cody, M.D., *Visualizing Muscles.* Lawrence, Kans.: University of Kansas Press, 1990.

William R. Hensyl, ed., *Stedman's Medical Dictionary,* 25th ed. Baltimore: Williams & Wilkins, 1990.

Fritz Kahn, M.D., "Man," in *Structure and Function,* vol. 1, translated and edited by George Rosen, M.D. New York: Alfred A. Knopf, 1947.

Eldera Pearl Solomon, Richard R. Shmidt, and Pete James Adragna, *Human Anatomy and Physiology,* 2nd ed. New York: Saunders College Publishers, 1990.

The oldest known ancestor who shared our basic modern musculoskeletal system, particularly the structures that enable upright posture and bipedal locomotion, is Lucy, an australopithecine fossil discovered in 1974 in East Africa. I use her age, approximately 3.2 million years, in this chapter and elsewhere to establish the longevity of the human musculoskeletal legacy. Lucy's importance is reported in Luigi Luca Cavalli-Sforza and Francesco Cavalli-Sforza, *The Great Human Diasporas,* translated from the Italian by Sarah Thorne. New York: Addison Wesley Publishing Co., 1995.

The statistics regarding the total number of chronic pain sufferers in the United States are from Shannon Brownlee and Joannie M. Schrof, "The Quality of Mercy," *U.S. News & World Report,* March 17, 1997.

The "diseases of civilization," the related quotation, and other material on pages 11 to 14 are drawn from René Dubos, *So Human an Animal.* New York: Charles Scribner's Sons, 1968.

Chapter Three

The Stanford University study referred to on page 36 was reported on the Internet by Yahoo News, "Bulging Disk Not Always Serious," Reuters Ltd., 1997.

A useful and important discussion of the danger of misconstruing lack of pain with good health is found in Norman Cousins's *Head First: The Biology of Hope and the Healing Power of the Human Spirit.* New York: Penguin Books, 1989.

Chapter Five

Data on the ankle's articulating surface and loading-impact stress come from Jürgen Weineck, *Functional Anatomy in Sports,* 2nd ed., translated from the German by Thomas J. DeKornfeld. St. Louis: Mosby–Year Book, 1990.

Chapter Seven

The concept of man as a "centaurlike" creature is offered by Colin Tudge, *The Time Before History.* New York: Touchstone, 1996.

Data on the condition known as *coxa valga* and on the hip's loading-impact stress come from Weineck, *Functional Anatomy.*

Information on clinical studies involving the benefits of moderate exercise in the abatement of arthritis pain is drawn from "Exercise—A Safe and Effective New Treatment for Knee Osteoarthritis," National Institutes of Health news release, December 31, 1996.

Chapter Eight

The metaphor of a jelly doughnut leaking its filling to describe a disk herniation is widely used by musculoskeletal specialists. It has been published by Joseph Kandel, M.D. and David B. Sudderth, M.D., *Back Pain: What Works*. Rocklin, Calif.: Prima Publishing, 1996.

A study of treatment outcomes for acute low back pain for various health care specialists, "The Outcomes and Costs of Care for Acute Low Back Pain Among Patients Seen by Primary Care Practitioners, Chiropractors, and Orthopedic Surgeons," was published as an Internet abstract of a special article by the *New England Journal of Medicine*, vol. 33, no. 14, October 5, 1995.

Chapter Nine

My use of triangles to describe the structural interaction of the torso owes a debt to chiropractor Wallace L. King's *The Spinal Tetrahedron*. Grand Forks, N.D.: Morgan Publishing Co., 1991.

Chapter Ten

For the operation of the radius and ulna and the muscles of the hand and wrist, it was helpful to consult Stephen Goldberg, M.D., *Clinical Anatomy Made Ridiculously Simple*. Miami: Medmaster, 1990.

Chapter Twelve

The figures pertaining to the predominant lack of regular physical activity by Americans and the rate of injury among runners comes from "Exercise for Women," editorial, *New England Journal of Medicine,* vol. 334, no. 20, March 16, 1996.

The flippant but apt term *StairMaster Butt* is from Jake Tapper, "Bummed Out on the StairMaster," *Washington Post*, March 19, 1997.

INDEX

ABOUT THE AUTHORS

Pete Egoscue, an anatomical physiologist, has been practicing his method since 1978. He runs the Egoscue Method Clinic in San Diego and is the author of *The Egoscue Method of Health Through Motion.*

Roger Gittines is a freelance writer living in Washington, D.C.